Case Studies in Communication and Disenfranchisement

Applications to Social Health Issues

LEA'S COMMUNICATION SERIES
Jennings Bryant/Dolf Zillmann, General Editors

Selected titles in Applied Communication (Teresa L. Thompson, Advisory Editor) include:

Cissna • Applied Communication in the 21st Century

Morris/Chenail • The Talk of the Clinic: Explorations in the Analysis of Medical and Therapeutic Discourse

Nussbaum/Coupland • Handbook of Communication and Aging Research

Ray • Case Studies in Health Communication

Ray • Communication and Disenfranchisement: Social Health Issues and Implications

Ray • Case Studies in Communication and Disenfranchisement: Applications to Social Health Issues

For a complete list of other titles in LEA's Communication Series, please contact Lawrence Erlbaum Associates, Publishers

Case Studies in Communication and Disenfranchisement

Applications to Social Health Issues

Edited by
Eileen Berlin Ray
Cleveland State University

LEA LAWRENCE ERLBAUM ASSOCIATES, PUBLISHERS
1996 Mahwah, New Jersey

Lawrence Erlbaum Associates, Inc., Publishers
10 Industrial Avenue
Mahwah, New Jersey 07430

Cover design by Gail Silverman

Library of Congress Cataloging-in-Publication Data

Case studies in communication and disenfranchisement : applications to social health issues / edited by Eileen Berlin Ray.
p. cm.
Includes bibliographical references and index.
ISBN 0-8058-1674-7 (c : alk. paper). — ISBN 0-8058-1675-5 (pbk. : alk. paper).
1. Marginality, Social—United States—Case studies. 2. Socially handicapped—United States—Case studies. 3. Victims—United States—Case studies. 4. Communication in medicine—United States—Case studies. 5. Social medicine—United States—Case studies.
I. Ray, Eileen Berlin.
HN90.M26C37 1996
306.4'61—dc20 96-823
CIP

Books published by Lawrence Erlbaum Associates are printed on acid-free paper, and their bindings are chosen for strength and durability.

Printed in the United States of America
10 9 8 7 6 5 4 3 2 1

To George, Janet, and Laurie
And to Aunt Lil

Contents

II ISSUES RELATED TO FAMILY

III ISSUES RELATED TO ABUSE

IV ISSUES RELATED TO HEALTH CONCERNS

Contributors

Terrance L. Albrecht
Department of Communication/
Family Health
College of Public Health
University of South Florida
Tampa, FL 33612

Sara Alemán
School of Social Work
Arizona State University West
Phoenix, AZ 85069

Fredi Avalos-C'deBaca
School of Communication
San Diego State University
San Diego, CA 92182

Deborah S. Ballard-Reisch
Department of Communication
University of Nevada, Reno
Reno, NV 89557

Mark Bergstrom
Department of Communication
University of Utah
Salt Lake City, UT 84112

Dawn O. Braithwaite
Department of Communication Studies
Arizona State University West
Phoenix, AZ 85069

Robin P. Clair
Department of Communication
Purdue University
West Lafayette, IN 47907

Rebecca J. Welch Cline
Department of Communication
Processes & Disorders
University of Florida
Gainesville, FL 32611

Frederick C. Corey
Department of Communication
Arizona State University
Phoenix, AZ 85287

Lynette Seccombe Eastland
Department of Speech
& Communication Studies
Clemson University
Clemson, SC 29634-1505

Patricia Geist
School of Communication
San Diego State University
San Diego, CA 92182

Julie L. Gray
School of Communication
San Diego State University
San Diego, CA 92182

Timothy J. Hack
Lafayette, IN

Ginger Hill
School of Communication
San Diego State University
San Diego, CA 92182

Gerianne M. Johnson
Department of Speech
& Communication
San Francisco State University
San Francisco, CA 94132

Daniel P. Joyce
Cleveland Mediation Center
Cleveland, Ohio

John Kahler
Department of Family Practice
Cook County Hospital and
Humana Health Care Plans
Chicago, IL 60615

Lisa Kanae
Department of Communication
University of Hawaii
Honolulu, HI 96822

Melissa Lavitt
School of Social Work
Arizona State University West
Phoenix, AZ 85069

Heather Manns
Department of Communication
Illinois State University
Normal, IL 61761

Alicia A. Marshall
Department of Speech Communication
Texas A&M University
College Station, TX 77843

Nelya J. McKenzie
Department of Communication
Auburn University at Montgomery
Montgomery, AL 36117

Janet K. McKeon
Department of Communication
Michigan State University
East Lansing, MI 48824

Sandra Metts
Department of Communication
Illinois State University
Normal, IL 61761

Katherine Miller
Department of Communication Studies
University of Kansas
Lawrence, KS 66045

Jon F. Nussbaum
Department of Communication
University of Oklahoma
Norman, OK 73019

Jennifer Price
Lakeland, FL

Eileen Berlin Ray
Department of Communication
Cleveland State University
Cleveland, OH 44115

Jill E. Rudd
Department of Communication
Cleveland State University
Cleveland, OH 44115

David R. Seibold
Department of Communication
University of California, Santa Barbara
Santa Barbara, CA 93106

Barbara F. Sharf
Department of Medical Education
University of Illinois at Chicago
Chicago, IL 60612

Lisa Sparks
Department of Communication
University of Oklahoma
Norman, OK 73019

Richard W. Thomas
Department of Speech
Communication & Dramatic Arts
Central Michigan University
Mount Pleasant, MI 48859

Teresa L. Thompson
Department of Communication
University of Dayton
Dayton, OH 45469

James T. West
Honolulu, HI 96822

Introduction

Eileen Berlin Ray
Cleveland State University

This book tells the stories of some of the disenfranchised in the United States. Each case focuses on aspects of how the communication–disenfranchisement relationship is accomplished, managed, and overcome. Through interactions with significant others, institutions, and the mass media, each person's place in American society is defined in terms of permissible identities, behaviors, topics of discussion, and expectations. In addition, this interaction clarifies who controls the resources, who makes the decisions, and who sets the social standards.

Each of us, if not at the present, is likely to become a member of one or more disenfranchised groups at some point in our lives. Whether for ourselves or someone we care about, we have been or will be impacted by these issues, leaving those not currently affected only "temporarily enfranchised." Thus, for some these stories speak to their past, to others their present, and to others possibly their future. The fact that we are all vulnerable adds to their poignancy and is further underscored by the case study format.

Case studies are a particularly useful method for making the abstract concrete. By merging theory and application (Ray, 1993; Sypher, 1990), they personalize important issues and enable us to more clearly visualize the complexities of a variety of interrelationships. However, although case studies alone are useful pedagogic tools, they are even more effective when directly tied to the theoretic considerations they are exemplifying. This volume was conceived of as a companion text to *Communication and Disenfranchisement: Social Health Issues and Implications* (Ray, 1996). By offering case studies that correspond to those chapters, the books used together provide a theoretically based application of social health issues within a communication framework.

The stories found in this book are told from a variety of perspectives. Some follow the personal story of the author, from the gay man's caring for his lover through his terminal illness (Corey, chapter 13), to the recalling of an adolescent's battle with cancer (Ballard-Reisch & Price, chapter 6), to a woman leaving an abusive marriage (Kanae & West, chapter 11). Some, by telling their stories through the voices of composite others, enable us to hear from, for example, the homeless (Miller, chapter 2), adult incest survivors (Ray, chapter 10), the sexually harassed (Hack & Clair, chapter 12), impoverished women (Marshall & McKeon, chapter 4), and the elderly (Nussbaum, Sparks, & Bergstrom, chapter 8). Others draw from the words of interviewees, such as persons with HIV/AIDS (Metts & Manns, chapter 14) or those involved in a major political battle against homosexuals (Eastland, chapter 1). Whatever the format, all provide powerful accounts of the experiences, challenges, and accomplishments of many of the disenfranchised.

Although the cases in this volume are not all-inclusive, they cover a breadth of issues and legitimize the relationship between communication and social health issues. As the field of health communication has continued to grow since the mid-1970s, research has primarily been restricted to examining the communication–physical health relationship (Ray, 1993). As a result, there has been significant inquiry into caregiver–recipient communication, health care organizations, health promotion campaigns, and health education. One outcome of this work has been a depth of knowledge in these areas. Another outcome has been the inadvertent drawing of an imaginary but strong boundary around what falls under the rubric of health communication. This boundary has led to unintentional academic myopia by making topics inside it salient and essentially marginalizing other relevant topics. As a result, although we have gained depth we have sacrificed breadth. Expanding the boundary to consciously include topics that have previously been ignored or stigmatized invigorates our research agenda, expands what "fits" within the health communication domain, and most importantly, will provide a more complete understanding of the communication–health relationship.

ORGANIZATION OF THE BOOK

The organization of this book parallels that of *Communication and Disenfranchisement: Social Health Issues and Implications*.[1] Part I examines how disenfranchisement and empowerment are communicatively affected

[1]The first three chapters of *Communication and Disenfranchisement: Social Health Issues and Implications* emphasize specific conceptual orientations and do not have parallel case studies. In this book, the case study corresponding to Eastland's chapter is included in Part I: Issues Related to Politics and Socioeconomic Status. Also, the chapter by Zambrana does not have an equivalent case study.

in a political campaign and because of socioeconomic status. In chapter 1 (Eastland), a gay male and a lesbian, both from conservative Christian backgrounds, describe their struggle with managing their identities as an ultraconservative/religious right-wing group (the Oregon Citizens Alliance) attempts to pass a state constitutional amendment denying homosexuals their civil rights. Within the context of a campaign that hoped to further disenfranchise gay males and lesbians, both reflect on the struggles, challenges, and support that have enabled them to resolve issues related to their sexual orientation and identity and their recognition of the importance of political empowerment. Miller (chapter 2) provides perspectives on homelessness from the domiciled, the undomiciled, and service providers. From the man who became homeless after construction jobs dried up and now feels comfortable living that way, to a 7-year-old girl now living in a shelter with her two brothers and mother after leaving a physically abusive marriage, to the man who was discharged from a psychiatric hospital and now spends his nights in the park or a shelter, to the formerly homeless family who were able, through help at a shelter, to get back on their feet, we gain insight into how marginalization of the homeless is affected by each person's personal experiences, biases, self-interest, world view, and/or occupation. In chapter 3, Kahler and Sharf apply and expand their Culturally Sensitive Model of patient–physician communication in the case of a child being treated for AIDS in an inner-city clinic. They show how just relying on the physician's technical expertise further disenfranchises patients and their families and suggest the family genogram as a method to elicit more complete information. By personalizing patients and their families and understanding their life circumstances, physicians can offer more useful and realistic care and help families become part of the health care franchise. Marshall and McKeon (chapter 4) follow an impoverished woman as she seeks information and treatment for a lump in her breast. As the woman, her family, and friends gather information, it becomes clear that they have been talked *at*, not *with*, regarding preventive health behaviors. The importance of involving the target audience in the dissemination of health-related information is emphasized by the fact that women in this neighborhood do not have potentially lifesaving information about breast cancer and are not aware of resources available in their community.

In Part II, cases focus on the communicative process of disenfranchisement in family settings. Chapter 5 (Avalos-C'deBaca, Geist, Gray, & Hill) focuses on the experiences of an infertile couple. While attending a friend's baby shower, they recall the many disenfranchising messages they received from friends, family, the medical establishment, and society when they were trying to conceive and the impact of these messages on the choices they made. From her experience, the woman hopes to counter these messages through her support for a friend now in the same situation. Ballard-Reisch and Price (chapter 6) share their family's experience when Jennifer (the second author) was diagnosed with leukemia at the age of 15. From diagnosis to treatment to recovery, they tell the story of their family's pain, stress, and strength through the eyes of their parents and Jennifer. From their different needs for seeking information to their lack of involvement in decision making to interactions with medical personnel, family, and friends, they recount enfranchising and marginalizing messages that affected them during this crisis. Chapter 7 (Rudd & Joyce) focuses on the dissolution of a couple's marriage. Using divorce mediation rather than the traditional adversarial divorce process, the couple work to improve their communication as they try to agree on their division of assets and child custody. Although the goal of mediation is to balance power inequities, it is clear that the role of the mediator is critical to ensure the power balance and not allow the couple's hurt, anger, and stereotypic roles to interfere with their negotiations. In chapter 8, Nussbaum, Sparks, and Bergstrom track the varied lifestyles and paths of aging taken by the five adult children of Italian immigrants. The realities of differences in their family and friend support networks, each one's physical health, and their living situation impact the adjustments they must make as they struggle with personal losses and try, in their individual ways, to remain a part of mainstream society.

Part III examines issues related to sexual and physical abuse of women. Alemán and Lavitt (chapter 9) take a feminist perspective to rape by recognizing the political context in which sexual violence occurs and is perpetuated in American culture. Following a rape scenario, they describe three versions of outcomes for the victim and discuss how the interrelationships of gender, class, ethnicity, and power affect the outcomes for the victim and rapist, as well as our interpretation of the events. Considered from a feminist framework, it is evident how rape victims are either empowered or further disenfranchised within each context. Ray (chapter 10) continues the subject of sexual abuse by examining salient issues for adult survivors of incest. In the context of a day-long survivors' retreat, the women's individual and collective voices are heard as they struggle with the aftereffects of their abuse on their lives and those they care about. The powerful stigmatizing messages from their perpetrator, some family members and friends, and society are challenged as they share their secret and develop a collective voice. Kanae and West (chapter 11) poignantly tell the first author's story of her physically and emotionally abusive relationship and her decision to leave her marriage. The authors discuss warning signs during Kanae's courtship, the confusion and fear she experienced as a battered wife, her isolation and dependency, and the turning point that gave her the courage to break away and start a new life. In chapter 12, Hack and Clair describe a professional woman's experience of sexual harassment by her boss. They highlight the self-stigmatizing messages as victims tend to blame themselves and the importance of support networks as those who are sexually harassed weigh the repercussions of each choice of action available to them.

In Part IV, issues related to physical health concerns are emphasized. Corey, in chapter 13, tells the story of the illness and death of his partner from cancer. Efforts to keep them disenfranchised, both as gay men and as persons dealing with a terminal illness, are underscored in their power battles with the partner's doctor and the willingness of the medical establishment to conterminously construct gay men and HIV disease. Metts and Manns (chapter 14) base their case on interviews they conducted with persons who have HIV/AIDS. Interviewees share how they felt when they discovered they were HIV+, how significant others reacted to their diagnosis, and their coping strategies. Their stories tell about their problems, their resourcefulness, their commonalities, and their diversity. Perhaps most inspiring is that while many have lost social support, their good health, and their attachments to others, their spirit remains strong. Cline and McKenzie (chapter 15) continue the discussion on HIV/AIDS, focusing on women. These women are stigmatized not only because of their illness but because they are women, and often women of color. As with the interviewees in Metts and Manns' case, the responses of two women to their HIV/AIDS diagnosis and their dilemmas unique to being women emphasize the individuality of each person's experience and the multiple societal messages that perpetuate their stigmatization.

In chapter 16, Thompson follows one woman's sudden illness and its impact on herself, her family, and her friends. Her previously strong relationships tend to remain strong whereas already troubled ones become more difficult. As her illness progresses, it becomes clear that the types, sources, and helpfulness of communication and support received by the patient and her family change as her illness advances until her death. Thomas and Seibold (chapter 17) explore alcohol abuse in the context of the workplace. Using a transactional perspective, they examine the interpersonal and sequential communication attempts to intervene when a member's drinking threatens the completion of an engineer team's project. As a result of his drinking, the alcoholic isolates himself from potential social support and the team excludes him from the project because of his irresponsibility and poor work.

Chapters 18 and 19 focus on issues related to persons with disabilities. Johnson and Albrecht (chapter 18) emphasize employment concerns for the permanently and temporarily disabled in the setting of a weekly meeting of the Job Finders Club. In addition to providing a place for social support, the meetings also enable persons with disabilities to share information and experiences. In this meeting, members discuss their responsibility to increase employers' recognition of, and sensitivity to, their needs and their legal rights under the Americans With Disabilities Act. By educating themselves and others, they can challenge others' misperceptions and promote changes in the workplace. Braithwaite (chapter 19) focuses on the importance of persons with disabilities being treated as "persons first." Through three scenarios, she examines disability as a health issue, as a social stigma, and as a culture. From a cultural perspective, adjusting to a disability is analogous to assimilating into a different culture. Once individuals are able to successfully assimilate, they can take the initiative and communicatively create, rather than react to, their desired impression of themselves. In this way, they can confront the stigmatization of others and enfranchise themselves.

The case studies in this book personalize some of the complexities of the communication–disenfranchisement relationship. Whether based on personal accounts, composites, or interview data, they provide a useful instructional tool. Within the classroom, case studies can be used to generate class discussion, in conjunction with some specific task, as an innovative method for presenting analyses, and as a basis for essay questions on exams (Miller, Mattson, & Stage, 1995). At a more personal level, they provide a vehicle for personal reflection, gaining insight and understanding unattainable from other methods, and reinforcing the need for social action. It should be noted that many of the cases deal with very personal issues and there is a strong likelihood that some students in any class have had personal experience with one or more of the topics. Although the cases are likely to provide validation and empathy for these students, they may also make difficult emotional issues salient. It is important to recognize that, even if asked, students may be unwilling to acknowledge or disclose this information. Therefore, instructors should be sensitive to these concerns and provide appropriate safeguards for these students.

All of the cases included in this book explore how disenfranchisement is communicatively established, controlled, and challenged. Used alone or in conjunction with the other text, this book contributes to expanding what is included under the academic umbrella of health communication. It is my hope that these cases will generate discussion among students, professionals, and academics and lead us to further expand our domain of inquiry.

ACKNOWLEDGMENTS

Much of the work on this book was completed while I was on sabbatical in the Education Centre at Lincoln University, Canterbury, New Zealand. I am extremely grateful to Neil Fleming, the director of the Centre, for his enthusiastic support and for providing financial resources. I want to acknowledge other members of the Centre, Ruth Margerison, Nicola Cameron,

Jenny Lee, and Carrie Moore for providing an ideal work environment and Paul Humphreys for proofreading manuscript drafts.

I greatly appreciate Kathy Miller's support and helpful comments during various stages of this project, the help from Kathleen O'Malley, Barbara Wieghaus, Sharon Levy, Amy Olener and the staff at Lawrence Erlbaum Associates throughout my work on this book, and Amy Capwell for her help with the author index. Thanks also to Janet Goodman for her wit and wisdom, which seem to follow me wherever I go. Finally, this project could not have been completed without the love, support, and humor of my family. I am especially grateful to my husband, George, for his remarkable ability to remain unflappable and to our daughter, Lesley, and our son, Bryan, for insisting that their voices be heard.

REFERENCES

Miller, K. I., Mattson, M., & Stage, C. (1995). *Instructor's manual for organizational communication: Approaches and processes*. Belmont, CA: Wadsworth.

Ray, E. B. (Ed.). (1993). Introduction. In E. B. Ray (Ed.), *Case studies in health communication* (pp. xv–xx). Hillsdale, NJ: Lawrence Erlbaum Associates.

Ray, E. B. (Ed.). (1996). *Communication and disenfranchisement: Social health issues and implications*. Mahwah, NJ: Lawrence Erlbaum Associates.

Sypher, B. D. (1990). Introduction. In B. D. Sypher (Ed.), *Case studies in organizational communication* (pp. 1–13). New York: Guilford.

PART I

ISSUES RELATED TO POLITICS AND SOCIOECONOMIC STATUS

1 *Defending Identity: Courage and Compromise in Radical Right Contexts*

Lynette Seccombe Eastland
Clemson University

> *In the postmodern world there is no individual essence to which one remains true or committed. One's identity is continuously emergent, re-informed, and redirected as one moves through the sea of ever-changing relationships. In the case of "Who am I?" it is a teeming world of provisional possibilities.*
>
> —Gergen (1991, p. 139)

The crowd clasps hands and slowly begins to sway back and forth together to the music, "We are gay and straight together and we are fighting, fighting for our lives . . ." Many eyes are filled with tears and here and there someone breaks down sobbing; others have expressions of resolve. In some way, everyone is touched. This rally is one of many held in Portland, Oregon, during the past 6 years as the cultural war against gay men and lesbians rages. Although there are no bombed out buildings from this war and only sporadic physical violence, there are still thousands of "war stories." Wars of "meaning" and "identity" can be every bit as violent as wars of might.

Included in this case study are two of those war stories, those of one gay man in his 50s and one lesbian in her late 40s.[1] Both have a conservative

[1]Because the campaigns are conducted under the cloak of conservative Christianity and because the major efforts at reform are tied in with Christian teachings, I have chosen to focus on the personal struggles of individuals who have or had some tie to conservative religious groups.

Christian background. One has sought to retain his Christian roots and still sees himself as a Christian; the other abandoned those beliefs long ago and today defines her spirituality in new and different terms. Both have struggled with the current campaigns and involved themselves in ways that are comfortable for them. Their efforts to cope in a somewhat hostile climate, while others define their experience in terms of their own beliefs, reveal both (a) ways in which they are able to empower themselves, and (b) ways in which the current campaigns against homosexuals keep them a stigmatized and disenfranchised group.

Jim Briones

> We're all on a spiritual journey and we need to accept people where they are in their spiritual journey whether we like where they are or not. None of us has arrived.

> Gay people are very spiritual people, but from what they see in the scriptures, you can't be gay and be a Christian—it's an oxymoron.

Jim is an HIV-positive gay man in his 50s and an artist. He is also a Christian. The recent antihomosexual campaigns are in some ways a metaphor for the ways in which Jim and thousands of other gay men and lesbians have been dealing with themselves for most of their lives. For them, the struggle over identity is one they have waged internally for a long time. Although for some the internal battle has quieted or resolved itself, for others it still goes on. It is not an issue that is ever likely to be fully resolved. As young gay men and lesbians reach adolescence and find who they are conflicting with the ways in which their families, their churches, and their local communities see them, the struggle will continue. For many young people this may end in suicide, because the suicide rate for gay teens is many times the national average. "This campaign," says Jim, "is like hitting us at, what for some of us, is our weakest point—who we are in relation to the rest of the world. Some of us struggle with that for our whole lives."

In the bedroom over his bed, Jim has hung a piece of his own artwork. It features a large red circle in which is printed in block capital letters the word *hate* with a large red slash over it. Painted fluidly in luminous white over this "no hating" sign is the word *love*, also in block capital letters. This simple message is a reflection of the way in which Jim has responded to the campaign. "It disturbs me to see the gay community reacting to the hate with more hate. We have to realize that they are just at a different place in their journey than we are."

Many gay men and lesbians begin to see themselves as most problematic as they come up against others' expectations. There is a sense of always somehow experiencing oneself as a disappointment to others. This creates an inner struggle with identity that can be both devastating and clarifying. This has been true for Jim and has happened in several contexts:

> I had been struggling with this for a long time, dating girls, and they always thought that I was, uh, special because I didn't try to take advantage of them and I won their hearts like that because I was so polite and kind. My mom told me I was leading girls on. Well, I like girls, ya know, some of my best friends are girls. Even now, as I'm gay, lesbians and other women are some of my best friends, confidants and um, so, I wasn't leading them on, but I came to realize that they thought I was leading them on because I was so nice—we'd go places together and have a good time . . . to them, I was just a super neat Christian man.

Jim's enjoyment of friendships with women became difficult to deal with when a close friend misunderstood his attentions and suggested he make efforts to change himself. "It was in the early 80s that a woman friend of mine asked me where I went to church and I was going to the Metropolitan Community Church (a gay church) at the time . . . and she was in love with me and she had seen something about the church on TV and she came to me in tears and said, 'Are you gay?' and it just hit her like a sledge hammer."

While in the military in the late 1960s, Jim had several relationships with men that were actively sexual, but still didn't think of himself as homosexual and made several attempts to date women. After the rigid structure of the military in which his relationships were clearly contained, Jim went through a period of several years where he attempted to ignore his "problem." "I knew that the feelings that I had were wrong, or at least that's the way I felt at the time, and that I had to suppress them and so I kept myself busy from the time I woke up until I went to sleep, being active." Jim opened a store and worked hard at making it profitable but found several years later that it wasn't going to work in a business sense. During this time Jim was an active Christian and met lots of wonderful people. "I had a few gay things happen, like I fell in love with a man at my church and, ya know, really grappled with that."

As time went on, Jim found it more and more difficult to deny who he felt he really was. He saw it as an either–or choice—a Christian or a homosexual. "I was always taught that in the Scriptures, it's not only what you do, but what you think and I believe that's true to a degree, and so I knew what my thought life was." He was hearing more and more about the gay life and it really tempted him to explore. After thinking things over he decided he had been denying his identity on several levels. Not only was he denying his sexual identity, he was denying himself as an artist. He had trained for 4 years at the Museum Art School and here he was sitting behind a desk doing a job he hated. Denying one part of yourself often means you are blind to other aspects of your identity. Other parts of himself had been pushed aside with the homosexual identity:

> So I quit my job, and decided to do artwork here at the house on a commission basis, and I tried very hard to understand who I was as a man, as a sexual being and I went to a bar . . . I came to the conclusion that if I was really all that bad, if I'd been, as the teaching goes, "given over to a reprobate mind," if He'd just given up on me, I might as well go out and do it up good, so . . .

During this time, Jim made an attempt to find a religious gay community to which he could relate. The gay churches he attended seemed to him to be places to meet others, but not places in which he felt he could explore "the deep questions" he was trying to deal with. "I couldn't get any answers there, so I stopped going." In retrospect, Jim says that he was so ingrained in the teachings that he wasn't able to see what other gay Christians he met tried to explain to him, that it was a matter of intent rather than sin. "I felt they were justifying it to be at peace within themselves. We all, as human beings, need to justify what we do to feel okay and I just couldn't do that."

Other men Jim has known have attempted to deal with their emerging identity in very different ways:

> There was a fellow I knew who was the son of a Baptist preacher who was gay and he struggled like I did for years and he finally decided, "I'm gay, I'm gonna go to New York, my folks won't know anything that's happening with me and I'll just go to school there forever," which he did. After ten years he came back. His lover had died of AIDS and he had turned into a very bitter person, completely divorced himself from the church and was involved in an extremely destructive lifestyle and I see that over and over again with people. I once dated a college student whose father was a Baptist seminary teacher. He was a musician with a Christian rock band. He put a rifle to his head and killed himself.

Jim finally decided to go "whole hog." He still went to church, was still a leader, and still taught Sunday school but became more actively homosexual. After going through a time he referred to as the "whore period," he settled back down and tried to keep himself from being totally in the gay lifestyle, knowing that he was a gay man and trying to reconcile it by going to church.

Jim has always been involved, in one way or another, as a Christian. After a stint in the service he was active in Youth For Christ leadership; later he became a deacon at church; now he finds his friends and spiritual sustenance through Dignity, a spiritual support group for gay and lesbian Catholics and their friends. The struggle began first inside himself—a jarring inconsistency between what he was feeling and what he had been taught. "I began to experience myself as problematic and the reason is that I was always taught that in the Scriptures, it's not only what you do, but what you think and I knew what my thought life was and it was contradictory to what I had been taught." So when the woman who was in love with him pointed him to an organization called Reconciliation, he began to attend. The organization, run by a formerly gay man and his wife, met at a local Baptist church. The ultimate aim of the group was "cure." "I thought, it can't hurt to go and if I can be cured that would be wonderful because it's a hard life and nobody in their right mind would choose it and if there was a way out, why not try it." Jim remembers what a struggle it was for some other members of the group. One friend had chosen a very different way of dealing with his problem:

> He married a woman who was old enough to be his mother. He wasn't sexually attracted to her, but he did love her as a person and this was his way of dealing with his gay issue. She became his person to be accountable to, who would help him in his struggle and he really loved her . . . None of his family went to the wedding, none of his gay friends except for me . . . and it was an extremely difficult time for him.

Jim's experience as a Christian has been punctuated with several difficult incidents, all at times when he has been most actively involved in church activities. The first was while he was serving as a deacon at the community church he had attended for many years. When asked to be an elder, Jim told his pastor of his sexual orientation and he and Jim decided that it would be a problem if it was revealed, but that as long as Jim wasn't actively involved with other men they could overlook it. When his orientation was brought to the attention of state and regional church authorities, he stepped down as elder and stopped attending the church. "I think church is a place for people to heal, not to create problems for one another, so I stopped going. I went to the elders and resigned and they were all touched by my story and what I had to say, except for one guy who just sat there." Jim points to this experience as one that has taught him not to judge others too quickly or too harshly. "He was a football player, a big macho guy and he wouldn't even look at me . . . everyone was hugging me and shaking my hand and wishing me well and telling me how much they thought of me. A couple days later I got this letter and it really touched me." Jim hands me a two-page letter written on lined notebook paper he has taken from the top of a stack of carefully preserved papers and articles he has assembled to show me. "The gist of it," says Jim, "is that I meant a lot to him and he wished me well." Jim was surprised by his reaction: "He was the only person who took time outside of the organization, to come to me and talk to me in a personal way." It is clear that giving up that church office was very difficult for Jim. The "discovery" of his homosexuality by members of his family has also changed his role as a spiritual leader in the family. He used to be the one that would say prayers at family meals but for several years his sister had jumped in and said the prayers. This past year that has changed and he is the one asked. Although his parents have been caring and supportive, they are still trying to "straighten" him out, and not all family members have been as open. So, he says, "they don't see me as a spiritual leader, I don't think, anymore."

A second incident occurred while Jim was working as art director for a Christian magazine. The magazine, a publication for families who teach their children at home, was more than just a workplace to Jim for several years. Jim explains and hands me a letter and photos from the pile of mementos on the table: "This was the family here. I keep this as a memento of what they thought about me and how I felt about them. We were a family for three years, and the little boy loved me like a brother and looked forward to my coming to work and we would walk together on breaks and stuff."

Jim shifts uncomfortably as he recalls the painful end to the association. During that third year he extended himself to a friend and his lover, who were having relationship problems. He sought cooperation from Jim in coercing his partner into staying in the relationship and when Jim refused, the young man threatened to notify Jim's employer of his sexual orientation. Jim set very clear boundaries and told him, "I can't be involved in this . . . I'm doing what I have to do, if that's the way you feel you have to handle it, then you do what you have to do."

Jim was sitting working at the computer when the call came into the office:

> He asked her, did she know that she had a homosexual working for her and that I was a homosexual. She turned around and covered the phone and asked me, "Are you homosexual?" I said, "Yes." She hung up and left the room to talk to her sister someplace out of town. They always decided together what they were going to do. She came back and told me that being gay or homosexual was okay, but that I needed to allow God to heal me, and was I willing to do that? By that time, I had been grappling, hoping that people would start to know I was gay so that I could start to really be who I was, and so, though it was scary and I didn't like it, I just halfway rejoiced that now I could just be who I am, and I said, "I'm gay and I'm a Christian

> and I feel that I can be. I'm loving, I don't abuse people . . ." And she said, "Well, we love you and we don't think we can allow you to be, to continue on in this lifestyle and us condoning it by letting you work here. We think that if you continue this way that you'll be lost forever, and so we need to help you see the situation you're in by letting you go and we'd like you to leave right now."

Jim offered to stay the rest of the evening and finish a deadline, but she refused his offer and said that if Jim was not going to repent and be open to God's healing, then he'd have to leave right then. He has not seen them since the incident. Somehow, Jim manages to make sense of it in a very forgiving way:

> I know it was difficult for them to do because I asked her if she'd had any feelings and she said for several years she'd kinda thought I was and it goes to show that in their hearts they didn't want to do what they felt they had to just like I didn't want to do what I felt like I had to do. We're all in a stage of denial in some way. So when it comes to the Christian right I see them as individuals. You can't paint them all with the same brush. There are people who are really sincere in their beliefs and, as much as they can, they are trying to be compassionate but they believe their teachings so strongly that they have to do some of the things they do.

Jim distinguishes between "genuine, thinking Christians" and ones whose faith is "all made up." A genuine Christian "is open to seeing evidence, they've got a mind, they're able to think, and they realize that life isn't as simple as a lot of people try to make it." He respects those who struggle with the issue and make decisions based on the "courage of their convictions," but he believes that for some Christians, the "don't ask, don't tell mentality" is simply a way to avoid having to think about and take responsibility for what you believe. "Nobody," he says, "wants to grapple with this. It's not pleasant and no matter what side you come down on it's not easy, so let's just avoid it and maybe it'll go away."

One way Jim has dealt with the ongoing campaign is to "come out" to his friends, family, and community. This is a route suggested by numerous gay and lesbian organizations and publications, and opted for by many community members. "I saw other people doing it and I saw that it really had an impact. People began to know who we were, so I took a great big breath and I wrote a letter to the editor and she called me and said, 'We're going to print your letter . . . and we'd like to have your point of view on how Measure 9 affects you.' " Jim showed me the article, "Gay Man Pleads Don't Judge Until You Know Me," printed beside one by a local fundamentalist preacher. He felt then that "coming out" was a matter of survival. "I was at a point that I had to do what I could do for myself and that's what I could do—let my friends and neighbors know that I'm gay; they know that I'm not the things the OCA [Oregon Citizens Alliance] was talking about." Jim has several examples, from among his friends, of others who took a similar route to contribute and cope. One woman, for example, who attended Dignity with Jim, wrote up a newsletter and sent it to all her friends and family. It explained who she was and about her relationship and life and included pictures.

Jim has written numerous letters to the editor during the campaigns. He enjoys writing but feels he needs to learn how to write effectively so that people will accept what he has to say. "I tend to get too emotional . . . I want to learn to write so that I don't turn people off. I felt like I was hysterical. My feelings at the time were that I was in the trenches. I was fighting for my life." He talks softly about his mood at certain times over the last few years. At first he planned to sell his house and move out of state if the initial measure passed. Now he feels that if the second measure passes he will contribute to help the resulting legal battles. He has realized, he says, that it isn't going away. It will continue to spread. He recalls a radio interview with some OCA supporters who were very open in discussing their intent to put people in office who would honor God's mandate and for them that meant "killing homosexuals." If we really understand the agenda of these people, Jim says, then "we will take this very seriously." The mood is such, he believes, that if there are laws against homosexuals, then violence against them is somehow okay.

Self-acceptance was difficult for Jim. "I had to start to accept myself as a valuable member of the community and that's not easy when you've been taught for years homosexuals are faggots, literally meaning they aren't worth anything except to be thrown on the fire to fuel the burning of the big logs. If you're taught that all your life, then you believe it and that's how you live your life."

The second statewide antihomosexual effort of the Oregon Citizen's Alliance was winding down at the time I interviewed Jim. Just a few weeks later the proposed measure, The Child Protection Act (Measure 13), was voted down and like many other gay and lesbian citizens of Oregon, Jim was emotionally worn out. A local community radio station (KBOO) had run a five-part series on the previous measure (Measure 9) on Coming Out Day. For Jim "it brought out all the issues and I just bawled my eyes out, all the pain, ya know. Just amazing."

Sandi Addison

> I won't have others telling me who I must be. That is my choice. R. D. Laing says that the Western world is mad, that we are preoccupied with control. That's what I see here, an effort to control not just what I do, but who I am.

Sandi's struggle has been very different from Jim's. Although once a fundamentalist and an aspiring preacher, she feels she came to a moment of truth. It was while she was working for an evangelical organization in Washington, DC, that she met and became involved with another woman. "It answered so many questions for me." She studies her hands while she talks. "At the time I would have denied it vehemently, but I think fundamentalism was an addiction for me." Sandi didn't go through the moral struggles some others have experienced; she left her obsession behind easily and didn't look back. "I think I was ripe for something new. I was disillusioned by the church. It was anti-intellectual and I thought God gave us our minds to use them." Today, Sandi's car sports two bumper stickers: "Fundamentalism is mind-death" and "My karma ran over my dogma." She credits the fundamentalist denomination to which she belonged with the deep identity crisis she experienced toward the end of her time as an active member:

> I can remember sitting on the floor in the library in Bible school in the psychology section and combing the books for some indication that it was okay, meaning Christian, to love yourself. I didn't love myself, and on some level I knew I was in real emotional trouble and that was the way out. I didn't really have an identity then. Being a lesbian had never even occurred to me, but I had learned the "God first, others second, and self last" lesson really well and I lost myself in the process. When I found a book about self-esteem, I was so relieved. I knew it meant a lot to me but I didn't know quite what to do with it. Later, when I began therapy, I was really angry. Meeting this woman became a way to explore myself and that made it extra compelling.

Sandi's struggle was about identity and self-esteem. It was not until about 20 years later that she began to explore her spirituality again. During that time she felt physically ill when she made any attempt to enter a church. She sees her time involved as a fundamentalist as a time during which a great violence was done to her. "While I was aware of an emptiness, I was not even a little open to returning to a traditional church setting. I had been badly damaged through that addiction. I had been through a recovery process, years of therapy, and returning to the church would have felt like returning to an abusive relationship." Then spirituality became popular and Sandi found a way to meet her spiritual needs through communal living, expanding awareness, and meditation. She belongs to a group of women who meet in various cities once or twice each year for a time of spiritual renewal and discussion and reads what she refers to as "new thought" literature voraciously:

> For me, the OCA campaign has raised some very old issues. Ones I thought I had settled but obviously still need to work on. OCA people were gathering signatures outside one of my favorite stores. It made me physically sick to walk past them and I felt like they were intruding into my life by being there.

> There were two brave young gay men holding signs on the other side of the entrance. They were clearly a little nervous and one or two shoppers had stopped to talk to them and lend support. I gave them a high sign and then lost it at the little old lady sitting at the OCA table. I told her she should be ashamed of herself; that she ought to take some responsibility for her actions and learn to think for herself. Later I knew that I had been yelling at a very old part of myself that I still haven't forgiven.

Sandi has faced the campaigns of the last few years and responded in ways she felt she could. She has "come out" to people at work, worn buttons, pasted bumper stickers on her car, posted a lawn sign, attended rallies, and written an article for a regional publication, but she has not worked in the organized campaign:

> It is such a volatile issue for me, I start to shake when confronted with it on the street, I react with anger and I don't like that and need to get past it before I feel okay dealing with it one-on-one. It feels like a real threat. From my perspective this very group of people once denied me my identity and now they are trying to do it to me again.

Sandi, in many respects, sees herself in the OCA supporters she encounters primarily on television or gathering petitions in front of stores. She wore her anti-OCA button for several weeks. Sometimes she would respond to the hate-stares in the stores by smiling; other times she would feel exhausted and numb. She found herself weighing where to shop by the attitude of the community in which the store was located, but even that was no guarantee. On rare occasions someone would thank her for wearing the button, or someone else with a button would meet her eyes and smile. She began to thank people who were wearing "straight but not narrow" buttons.

> It was like we were creating a community with our attitudes. In a crowd I would always search out those with like minds in a sort of psychic sense and we would hold on to each other against the hate. We didn't ever need to speak a word to each other, it just sort of happened. If I felt that I was alone surrounded by hostile people, I would somehow sense it and get scared.

In many ways, Sandi sees the basic premise behind the campaign as evidence of a dysfunctional approach to life. "It is simply a reflection of the refusal to take responsibility for what we believe, feel, and do."

In some ways, Sandi feels ambivalent about the emphasis in the campaign on male homosexuality. Although lesbianism is assumed to be included, it is clearly the male lifestyle that is focused on in OCA literature. Whereas this helps her detach some from the attacks, it also tells her that women are still second-class citizens. "Gee, even our *sin* doesn't count to these creeps."

Unlike many other lesbians, Sandi does not believe she was always a lesbian and waiting to realize it. She believes she could have gone on being heterosexual and been okay, but not very fulfilled by it. "Before this woman approached me, it never even occurred to me that such an option was out there. I hate it because my experience conforms to their 'proof' that homosexuals recruit and can lure others into the lifestyle." Because of this Sandi has reexamined her own lesbianism and sees herself as having made a choice, but a choice that is fully her own. "This is *my* experience and nobody else's business. I don't have a single other friend that sees their experience this way."

Regardless of how she came to her identity, Sandi never wavers in terms of being a lesbian, but the meanings for that twist and turn in each new light. During the early 1970s, she says, she sees herself as having been a political lesbian, a radical feminist, and separatist. "I have been trying to integrate more good men into my life. I know instinctively that is something that has to happen for me to grow spiritually, but it is hard because I haven't really had men in my life in any meaningful way before and I have a hard time understanding them." Ninety-nine percent of the time, Sandi says, she is very happy as a lesbian. "It is wonderful and supportive and a caring, nurturing community to be a part of." The other 1% of the time she spends angry.

CONCLUSION

The campaign of the conservative and religious right is an effort to render invisible those who they see as problematic. They aim to accomplish this by sponsoring and campaigning for ballot measures that: (a) explicitly recognize the "perverse" nature of homosexuality, (b) make explicit discussion of homosexuality in an educational setting illegal, unless it notes its "perverse" nature, and (c) remove any protections that exist against discrimination toward gay men and lesbians. In labeling homosexuality perverse, in crippling educational efforts about it, and in removing protection, the religious right hopes to drive gay men and lesbians back "into the closet." In addition, they sponsor and support reform programs to bring gay men and lesbians into a more "normal" lifestyle. This amounts to what Berger and Luckmann (1967) referred to as "conceptual liquidation," a process through which one group seeks to define another out of existence.[2]

[2]Conceptual liquidation is discussed by Berger and Luckmann (1967) in *The Social Construction of Reality* (pp. 108–115). A part of the conceptual machinery that maintains our universe, conceptual liquidation operates through therapeutic processes to keep everyone within the universe in question, and through processes of nihilation, to liquidate everything outside it. The process involves three components. First, there must be a central body of knowledge that includes a theory of deviance as constituting a threat to traditional modes of being. Second, there must be a way to account for the deviance (where does it come from?). Last, there must be a conceptual system for the "cure of souls," which operates to integrate the "deviant" back into society. In this case, the final step in conceptual liquidation involves "queer cures," programs that operate to help "sick" homosexuals escape the lifestyle.

The case studies presented here are aimed at providing an understanding of the impact of these campaigns on members of the disenfranchised group. Both Jim and Sandi have come to resolution in terms of their sexual orientation and identity. Both feel that there is much more to that identity than sexual behavior and Sandi makes it explicit that her sexuality is only one small part of who she is. Deciding who we are and defining our identity is a struggle for all of us but even more of a struggle for those whose identity is seen by some as a "problem."

RELEVANT CONCEPTS

conceptual liquidation
empowerment
personal control
"queer cures"
social construction of identity

DISCUSSION QUESTIONS

1. What practical suggestions for empowerment emerge out of Jim's and Sandi's struggles?

2. Sandi suggests that "control" is at the heart of the current cultural war over homosexuality. Discuss the ways in which control is relevant here.

3. Kenneth Gergen (1991), in *The Saturated Self,* contended that: "One's potentials are only realized because there are others to support and sustain them; one has an identity only because it is permitted by the social rituals of which one is part; one is allowed to be a certain kind of person because this sort of person is essential to the broader games of society." What are the broader "games of society" that are relevant in this case and how does conceptual liquidation play a part in them?

4. This case study begins with another quote by Gergen (1991). He sees the postmodern self as one that is anchorless and exists primarily in relation to others. Address this notion of the self in the cases of Jim and Sandi.

REFERENCES/SUGGESTED READING

Berger, P., & Luckmann, T. (1967). *The social construction of reality*. New York: Doubleday.

Gergen, K. (1991). *The saturated self: Dilemmas of identity in contemporary life*. New York: Basic Books.

Kitzinger, C. (1987). *The social construction of lesbianism*. London: Sage.

Shotter, J., & Gergen, K. (1989). *Texts of identity*. London: Sage.

2 *Conflicting Voices: Homelessness in America*[1]

Katherine Miller
University of Kansas

Practically everyone has heard the old legend about the blind men trying to describe an elephant. With each sightless explorer groping at a different portion of the beast, a listener would be hard-pressed to believe that all were describing the same animal. Homelessness is a lot like that. It can be described as a "social problem," an "urban plague," or a "choice," depending on who is addressing the issue. Causes for homelessness vary from bad luck to personal fault to the insidious creeping of the welfare state, depending on the point of view. Solutions seem obvious or unattainable, depending on the perspective. In the following pages, homelessness is considered from 10 perspectives that are unique, limited, and revealing. Let's listen in as four homeless people and six domiciled people talk about homelessness in today's America.

THE VOICE OF FATHER TIM

I used to think about homelessness in philosophical terms. I'd look at it as a social issue or a policy problem or even as a spiritual shortcoming. These days, I've given up on those philosophical meanderings and just

[1]This case is based on a multidisciplinary study of homelessness in the greater Phoenix area. It included interviews and surveys with homelessness service providers and volunteers and an ethnographic investigation of homeless individuals and families.

work to deal with homelessness on a day-to-day basis. You see, I run a shelter for homeless men and when you're that close to the problem, there isn't the time or the energy for abstract theorizing. There's only time for the minuscule details of daily life and the monumental tasks of sorting out bureaucratic red tape.

As part of our religious mission, we run a shelter called "Pathways." It's an emergency shelter for single men. We can house guys for up to 1 week, then we have to move them along to some kind of transitional housing program or to a different emergency shelter. Or, sadly, back to the streets. We provide a bed to sleep on and an evening meal, and try to help the guys out in other ways like mail service, showers, phones to use, health referrals, training options, and drug and alcohol programs. Of course, we can't do all those things for every man that comes through, and quite frankly, a lot of them just want to get out of the cold and rain for a few days. So we do what we can and try to not get discouraged.

There are a lot of homeless men, though, who never come near the shelter. There are too many rules and they feel robbed of their freedom and identity. The guys have to check in by 4:00 p.m., be in line for dinner by 5:00 p.m., lights out at 9:00 p.m., wake-up at 5:00 a.m., and out of the door by 6:00 a.m. Of course, no drugs or alcohol are allowed on the premises, and we only house single men—no women, no kids, no families. So it's not exactly a five-star resort, but it does provide some temporary help to people in need.

I wish I could do more for the guys. I wish I even had more time to spend talking to them—listen to their stories, hear about their problems. But there isn't much time for that. Instead, I'm caught up in the bureaucracy of running a shelter. First and foremost, I have to deal with daily issues of keeping Pathways moving. Getting dinner from the food bank. Having volunteers ready for the serving line. Keeping track of how many beds are filled. Referring women and families to other appropriate shelters. All of these things take up a great deal of time. But there are the bigger issues of making sure this place even survives. Dealing with the church bureaucracy. Applying for government grants. Coordinating activities with community groups. Gladhanding local politicians.

Do I sound frustrated? Sadly, I guess I am. I know I'm running this shelter for the right reasons, and I know the help I give these men is valuable in many ways. But dealing with a small portion of the "solution" to homelessness only makes me painfully aware of how the problem as a whole might be insoluble. At Pathways, we're addressing the symptoms, and that's a step in the right direction. But is it possible to fix the diseases that cause homelessness? Can we even put a finger on what those diseases are? Those are the questions I struggle with every day. And much to my dismay, I don't feel any closer to answers than I did when Pathways opened 8 years ago.

THE VOICE OF ZEKE

The street has been my home for almost 10 years now. I move around a lot. I spend most of my time around Texas—Houston, San Antonio, Austin. Sometimes I get over to New Mexico or Arizona and I've even spent some time in California. But I like Texas. I grew up here and it's a comfortable place for me.

I never really planned to be on the road for this long. I used to find pretty steady work in construction, but then jobs started to dry up. I began to move around to find more work, but it just wasn't there. Down on my luck, I was. And my parents died a long time ago, and there just wasn't anyone to stay with, so here I am. I don't look for construction work much anymore, though. I wouldn't want to get tied down to one spot or be responsible to anyone but myself. My life might not seem like much to you, but it's what I know and I'm not sure I could or would change it now. You've gotta respect a man's life, whatever it is.

Most people don't understand what life on the street is like. They don't want to understand. They turn their heads when they see us, walk on the other side of the road, or look right through us as if we're not there. I'm not saying that being treated that way doesn't hurt, but hey, you get used to it. They don't know my life, and there's no explaining it to someone who doesn't want to know. I don't just sit on the street all day. I've got activities, I've got things to do, I've got friends. So don't feel sorry for me, and most of all, don't pretend you know what's best for me.

I usually sleep on the street if it's warm or in an abandoned building if it's cold. I don't go to the shelters. They don't want to deal with people like me who have been around for a long time, and I don't want to deal with all the bullshit in the shelter. So I make do outside. Sometimes I'm alone, sometimes I've got buddies to hang out with at night. There are spots in every city where you can find a roof and guys to talk to at night. Usually at night we'll try to get a bottle or two to share. That's the great thing about guys on the street. They never have much of anything and might spend their last dollar on a bottle of wine. But then they'll share that wine with you. And they know that the next night, if I've picked up a few bucks, I'll bring the bottle.

During the day, there's a lot to keep me busy. I sometimes go down to the Salvation Army for breakfast, but that's done with by 7:30, so most of the time I don't make it. But there are other places you can get a cheap bite to eat and unlimited coffee in the morning, so some of us hang out together, look through the paper, and shoot the breeze. Then we've got to figure out ways to get some cash. Every few days, we can go to the plasma center, and some guys go down to the day labor center religiously. Others survive by panhandling, but I only do that as a last resort. Instead, I've figured out the best dumpsters in most towns for bottles and cans, and with some industrious gathering, I can make a few bucks every day on recycling. Then, there are the soup kitchens for lunch and dinner, or we'll go to a fast-food joint if we've got some cash. Then it's time to find a spot for the night, maybe get a bottle, and settle in. Sometimes we get hassled by the cops, especially if there are too many of us together, but we usually can just move on and no one bothers us too much.

This probably isn't the life you would choose for yourself. I'm not sure it's the life I would choose for myself. But it's the life I've got and it's not for anyone else but me to judge whether it's a good life or a bad life. Things might change. I figure I'm due for some good luck one of these days—I've certainly paid my dues. But in the meantime, I get by.

THE VOICE OF MEGHAN

My name is Meghan and I'm 7 years old. I have two little brothers. Nathan is 3 and Nicholas is 1. Nicholas and Nathan and me and my mommy all live in a shelter. I didn't used to tell anybody that I lived in a shelter, but we've been here for a while now, so I'm used to it. The shelter is an okay place. My mommy and brothers and me all have to sleep in the same room. It's kind of crowded, but that's okay. There are some other kids and other mommys here, too. We all eat together, and there's a room where we can watch television and there are toys and stuff for us to play with. I've made a new friend here, too. Her name is Haley and she's 7, just like me. Haley and me both go to the same school. We're in second grade together. I don't have a lot of friends there other than Haley. There are some girls who maybe would want to be my friend, but I don't want to tell them where I live. My friends used to come to my house and play, but now I don't have a house anymore. I don't want to tell kids I live in a shelter. My teacher knows, I think, but I don't want to tell anybody else. Haley doesn't tell anybody either.

Mommy and Nathan and Nicholas and me all used to live in a house with our daddy. It was nice that we were in a house and I had some friends to play with, but my mommy and daddy sometimes would fight. It made me sad. They'd yell at each other a lot, and sometimes my daddy would push my mommy. Then I think sometimes he would hit her, and I was scared of him, too. So after a while, my mommy said we were going to have to go away. One day, she helped me pack up my clothes and toys, then we both helped get Nicholas and Nathan's stuff together. Then we all left. We lived for a few days with my Aunt Jean, but there really wasn't room in her house for all of us plus Aunt Jean, Uncle Pete, and all my cousins. So we had to find another place to go. My mommy called someone on the telephone and then we came here. I don't know how long we've been here. It's been a while, but not as long as I had lived in my house before.

Mommy told me that pretty soon we are going to be able to live in another house like we used to before, but not with Daddy. There are people who are helping us to do that, but I think it's hard for Mommy. I think maybe she's going to have to find a job and find someone to help watch us, but she says it's hard to find a job and it costs money to have someone watch us. So for now we're all going to stay here in the shelter. Like I said, I guess that's okay, but a house would be better.

THE VOICE OF PAUL

My name is Paul Grayson. I own three jewelry stores in town. Started them up on my own 20 years ago, and I must say they're doing quite well. I'm also very active with the local Rotary and I'm president-elect of the Chamber of Commerce. People respect me and I work hard to make this community a pleasant and prosperous place to live.

You've asked me to tell you what I think about homelessness. I never used to think about homelessness at all, but I've had to lately, because it's getting out of hand here. There have always been a few vagrants here and there, but now there are lots more sleeping in the park and you see them on the streets quite a bit. They just put in a new soup kitchen down the block from one of my stores and it makes me furious. Those people loiter around the streets for hours around serving time, and my customers don't like to see that. I've had to talk to the director of the soup kitchen on numerous occasions about keeping her people contained to her building. There's been more litter since they moved in, and I'm even starting to worry about rats.

And now there are debates in City Council about building an additional shelter somewhere. Of course, the obvious spot would be down on Washington Street where all those people hang out. But some people want to build it at the edge of town or even in the suburb where I live. They don't want to have a ghetto, and think services should be spread out. I'm speaking up strongly against that. We don't have a homelessness problem in *my* part of town, and I don't want to get one by building a shelter. It's bad enough to have the area around Washington Park turning into an eyesore—it used to be a pleasant place to take the family on the weekend. But at least let's keep the problem from spreading beyond that area of the city.

I'm also worried, from a Chamber of Commerce point of view, about what the homelessness problem might mean for the city's economic future. We've started to recruit a lot of convention business. Our climate is attractive and we're getting the hotel base we need. But how are out-of-towners going to feel about seeing those people on the street or being followed and begged for money? I heard that in Miami they sometimes do "sweeps" to clean the homeless out of areas where there are a lot of tourists. I'm not saying that's the right solution, but we have to do something. We need to be sure that the city belongs to the people who work hard to maintain it and keep it strong. We need to deal with the situation before it gets any worse.

THE VOICE OF MARIA

I've got a pretty good life. Oh, I guess it wouldn't look like anything special to you. I've got three kids—Gloria, Adam, and Michael—they're 14, 10, and 8 years old. They're good kids. My husband, Joe, works for a small engineering firm. He likes his job and works real hard at it, and he makes enough money so that I don't need to work and we can still live comfortably. We've got a nice house with a nice yard, and the kids do sports in the afternoon and take music lessons. I work on PTA stuff and do the church newsletter. So it's a pretty normal life and we all like it.

But I think a lot about how lucky I am. Me and Joe are doing a lot better than either of our parents did, and we hope it turns out that way for the kids, too. But these days, there's nothing you can count on. The world has been good to us, but it can be a cruel place.

Maybe the reason I think so much about this stuff is that I've started working three afternoons a week at this soup kitchen run by the church. I first signed up to do the serving line one day after Mass and I've started working there pretty regularly in the last few months. I've been there so much that I'm a supervisor of other volunteers on the days I work. We get the food in from the food bank or from whatever group is helping out with food that day. It's never anything very fancy, but it's always filling and tastes okay. Then we get everything prepared and get the food line ready by 4:30 or so. Folks are lined up by then, so we usually start dinner right away. It's first come, first served, but everyone knows to be there pretty early and there's usually enough for everyone who's hungry.

As much as I can, I try to talk to folks. I sit down and eat with them if I can or chat with them while they're in line. Sometimes people don't want to talk, but once they know I'm not going to be judging them, they're usually glad to have someone different to chat with. I guess before I never really thought about the kind of people who had to go to a soup kitchen for dinner. If I did think about them, I figured they were people a whole lot different from me. Once you start hearing their stories, though, you realize that the people in that soup kitchen line are as different from each other as everyone else is. You can't just lump them into a pigeonhole labeled *homeless*. Some of them have real serious problems with alcohol or drugs. Some of them are probably mentally ill—or on the edge of it. Some of them are people who just ran out of money and can't get back on their feet. Sometimes families come by that aren't homeless, but can't afford to put food on the table so they come down every day to eat. They've all got their stories, they've all got their heartaches.

Some of my friends ask me why I keep volunteering and going downtown 3 days a week to do the cooking and serving. Some of them have gone once or twice, but they've gotten real uncomfortable. They don't look at the people as they're dishing up the food. They want to say they've helped, but they're scared. Maybe it's that "There but for the grace of God" kind of thing, or maybe they're just so far removed from that kind of life that they can't relate. I don't know. All I know is that for me, helping out at the kitchen has really opened my eyes. Now when they talk about homelessness on the news, I don't think of a bunch of people on park benches. Instead I think of Mr. Peabody, a confused old guy, but nice as can be. Or about Sam and Lisa and their two kids who have been living in their car since they moved out west. You see, the shelters won't allow the men to stay with the women and the children and they'd rather be outside than be separated. Or I think about Jack, a young guy trying to get over a drug problem and find some work. And I think about me, and Joe, and Gloria, and Adam, and Michael. And I remember how lucky we are.

THE VOICE OF GERIANNE

I've been a public health nurse for almost 20 years. I've done a lot of different kinds of work since getting out of nursing school. For a while I worked in the elementary schools, then I worked with a program that did follow-up work on premature and low-birth-weight babies. Both of those jobs were interesting and rewarding, but when I look back, they were pretty boring compared to what I do now. For the last 6 years, I've worked in a community outreach program that provides medical care to homeless people. It's a great program. There are only five employees—the program administrator, three nurses, and a social worker. And, there are several physicians who volunteer their time to the program. So we're stretched given the small staff, but we do what we can.

Our work mostly involves providing as much care as we can to people living on the streets. Sometimes it's preventive care like immunizations for kids, but most of the time it involves providing the immediate care necessary for both chronic and acute problems. For example, there are a lot of homeless folks with sexually transmitted diseases, and we do what we can to get them treatment. Or, there are assorted health problems associated with being outside all of the time—exposure problems in the winter, heat exhaustion in the summer, foot problems (from going without good shoes) almost all the time. Or with the kids, there are always the normal problems of ear infections and flu, plus more than the normal problems with things like upper respiratory disease, head lice, and stuff like that. So we've got our hands full most of the time.

There are a number of things that are really difficult about my job. The first is the problem of even finding the people who need care. We have a clinic on the street, but a lot of times the people that need our help don't know we're here, or they can't get here. So we do a lot of driving out to the areas of town where the homeless live and we provide care on site. It takes a lot of time, but those folks would never get any care otherwise. That's the saddest part of my job—to go out to near the farm fields or under the bridges and see the conditions under which people live. I know I'm doing what I can for them, but it breaks my heart to know that more isn't being done.

The second thing that's pretty frustrating about my work is all the paperwork that I have to deal with. Of course, the brunt of the paperwork falls on Carrie, our administrator. But I still have to fill out forms for every intake, and following these people can be a nightmare. They usually don't have proper identification, and we need to get pretty complete information in order to keep our funding. It just irks me that I have to spend so much time filling out forms when my training as a nurse is essentially going to waste.

The third thing that bugs me is the attitudes of a lot of other people about the homeless. Most of my "clients" have already been squashed by the system and, in my job, I often find myself watching them get squashed further. A lot of times we have to take people with chronic problems to the hospital or to other care providers. It's usually incredibly difficult to get help for them—they get ignored or talked to as if they're really stupid. It's like hospitals don't want someone who smells a little bit funny in their waiting room. And even if they get some help, I have to follow up every step of the way to make sure they get the continuing care they need. I understand that the homeless aren't "paying customers," but as far as I'm concerned there are some basic things that everyone deserves. They deserve to eat. They deserve to have someplace to sleep. And they deserve to be taken care of when they're sick. Everyone deserves those things, no matter who they are.

THE VOICE OF HAROLD

I've been alone for a long time. I don't have any family. I used to, but they're all gone now. My parents died long ago, and I've lost track of my two brothers. They might be dead now, too. I was never married, and never had any kids. So now that I'm getting pretty old, there's just me.

For most of my life, I lived in the hospital. I was home with my parents some when I was a kid, but I was sick even then. I'd hear voices telling me things, and parents and teachers would tell me that I was out of control. So sometimes when I was a kid they'd put me in the hospital when the voices got real bad. And when I got older, I was still in the hospital a lot, because the voices never really went away.

And that's the way it was for a long time. I'd be in the hospital, and I'd be feeling better with medication and with having doctors around to help me and talk to me. Sometimes I'd leave the hospital and go to a halfway house where I could cook my own meals and go on the bus downtown. But I'd usually have to go back to the hospital after a while. I never had a job that you could speak of. Just helping out folks with errands and chores and stuff like that.

Then, they told me I'd have to leave the hospital. I went to a group home to live for a while and was doing okay with my medicine, but then I was told that I had to leave the group home, too. There wasn't the money to keep me there, and they said I was well enough to leave the home. They had a big word for why I had to leave—government mumbo jumbo—but I don't remember what it was anymore.

So, now I live in the shelter sometimes, or in the park sometimes. I can still get my medicine if I go down to the clinic. They've got a list of people like me who get medicine. But I don't always remember, and if I forget then I get really confused and start hearing the voices again.

My friend, Jake, helps me out sometimes. He's a lot younger than me, but he kind of takes care of me. He'll get me to the shelter if I need to go there and he reminds me about my medicine. We usually go to the soup kitchen for meals together and he takes me to the clinic if I'm getting sick. It's good that I have a friend like Jake, now that I can't live in the hospital anymore. I hope he never has to leave me.

THE VOICE OF JULIE

You want to hear my story? I don't know that you really do, because, like, it's not a very pretty one. But, yeah, if you really want to hear about what's happened to me, I'll tell you. Where should I start? Well, I guess I'll just try to explain how I got to where I am now, sitting in this shelter with no money, nowhere to go, and a baby daughter to take care of.

I'm 21 years old now, but I guess I feel a lot older than that. I have a little girl, Natalie, who's almost 3. Would you like to see a picture of her? She's really cute. I think she looks like me but her hair's curlier. But back to my story. Anyway, when I was growing up, things weren't very good. We didn't have much money and my dad drank a lot. Sometimes he'd get after me and my brothers, and my mom never did much about it. She was just worn out, I guess. Anyway, I ran away the first time when I was 13 years old. I wasn't gone very long that time—it was cold and lonely and I didn't have any money so I went back home after a few days. But things never got any better around home. In fact, they got a lot worse. My dad drank more and my mom did less and less about it. My dad picked some on my little brothers, but mostly he picked on me. Sometimes it was yelling at me, sometimes it was hitting me, sometimes it was coming on to me. So I left again, finally for good, when I was 15. I didn't know where I was going to go, so I bought a bus ticket for L.A. I thought maybe I could get a job as a waitress or something and I had a little money saved for while I was looking for a job.

Then when I got to L.A., I couldn't find a job and I ran out of money pretty quick. I won't get into all the details, but to make a long story short, I ended up turning tricks on the street. For a while I tried working on my own, but that's tough, and eventually Jimmy got a hold of me and told me he'd take care of me. Having Jimmy around was kind of good and kind of bad. He protected me, but I was also scared of him. I belonged to him and I couldn't do nothing about it. It was like my dad again, sort of. I worked for Jimmy for a couple of years.

Then, I got pregnant. I think Natalie is Jimmy's kid, because all the customers always wore condoms. But Jimmy doesn't think she's his kid. Jimmy won't have anything to do with her—or with me either, for that matter. I'm not much use to him now, I guess. Anyway, after I got pregnant, I did find some work here and there waitressing. I made enough money to get by and lived with a couple of other girls who were trying to get off the street. I went to the free clinic to make sure I was okay with the baby and all. When I had her, I was so happy. She was the sweetest thing I ever saw and really a good baby.

But, good baby or bad, with a baby it's hard to work, so I had to quit my job. I got on AFDC and food stamps so me and Natalie could get by. But then the other girls I was living with didn't want a baby around, so Natalie and I had to move. There was this guy we knew who had a little apartment over his garage and he said we could live there. It was a pit, but the rent was free. We lived there for a while and were getting by okay on our monthly check. But then Hal started getting hassled about having someone live over his garage and he told us we had to find somewhere else. So we started looking.

Well, I couldn't find anyplace to live so I came to this shelter. It's a place to sleep, which is good. But the kicker is, now that I'm living in a shelter, I don't have an "address" like I did when I was living with the girls or living over Hal's garage. And when you don't have an address, you can't get government support. So now the AFDC payments have stopped coming in. And without the AFDC, I don't know that I'll ever be able to afford rent on even a piss-poor place like Hal's garage. So maybe me and Natalie are stuck here in this shelter. I don't know. I've got to get help, but I don't know quite how.

THE VOICE OF SYLVIA

My husband, Phil, says he doesn't believe in homelessness. Oh, he doesn't mean homelessness is like Santa Claus, like he doesn't believe homelessness *exists*. He just means that he doesn't believe in the "problem" of homelessness like you see on the television and read in the paper. He says that the liberals want us to feel sorry for the homeless, when sympathy is really the last thing those people need. What they really need—according to Phil—is the gumption to get a job and support themselves and their families the way most Americans do.

I'm not sure that I totally agree with everything Phil says on the topic, but, as usual, he has some good points. Maybe there are some homeless families who really have a difficult time finding work and supporting themselves. But you've got to wonder how hard most of them try. Every day I see homeless people panhandling on the street, or lined up at the plasma center, or standing at the entrance to the freeway with signs saying "Will work for food" or "Disabled vet—please help." Sometimes they're even standing there with children. When I see those people, I usually wonder how they got into the straits they're in. A lot of times I'm just too embarrassed to look at them. And sometimes I feel angry because I can look at those people and they look perfectly capable of finding a job without hankering on people like us. You'd think if they took the time to look over the want ads instead of begging, they could get out of trouble a lot faster.

I know it sounds shameful, but I really don't want to have to deal with those people every day. It's bad enough to have them chasing after you when you go downtown for lunch or the theater—I know I'll never get used to just ignoring them or flat-out refusing them. Anyways, it's one thing when they're downtown. It's quite another when I see them out in the area where I live. Phil and I worked hard to be able to afford a house here and we work hard to keep it up. Our kids go to good schools and we're instilling the kind of values we think will see them through life. What are they to think when there are scraggly bums hanging out just down the street from us?

Just listen to me. I sound like one of those suburban housewives who lives in a bubble. I'm not. I know how the world works and I know there are reasons for homelessness. But I also know this. There *are* jobs out there. There *are* ways to get help from your own family without counting on the government to bail you out. And people like me and Phil and our kids are entitled to live in a peaceful and quiet place without having to deal with those people every day. Maybe it sounds heartless, but those programs like AFDC and all those government grants aren't really helping these people. Grants and aid just give folks a crutch to lean on—a way to avoid the hard work of finding a job or finding a way to make it alone. And until those people learn that the government isn't going to be there with a handout every time they turn around, we're never going to be able to solve the problem.

THE VOICE OF NEAL

Me and my family used to be homeless. I've got a wife and four kids. Me and Sharla got married just out of high school and we had Jason right away. Then there was Jillian, then the twins—Corey and Kyle. So there we were, barely 25 years old, with four kids. When I was younger, I'd thought about going to college, but I never really had the grades for it, and then with us getting married and having the kids, well, I just had to get to work. For a while I had a steady job in a tool and die shop at the edge of town. But then when the car business got bad, I got laid off. I found some work with lawn maintenance places and other part-time stuff here and there, but it was never really enough to make ends meet. Sharla couldn't work—not with all the kids—so it was up to me.

Well, for a long time we managed to keep the kids fed and stay in the apartment we were in. Sometimes Sharla and me wouldn't have a lot to eat, and there were never a lot of toys or new clothes for the kids, but we got by. Then I fell off a ladder while I was trimming a tree and hurt my back. I couldn't do the lawn work anymore—couldn't do much of anything for a while. And we didn't have insurance, and there were medical bills to pay. Sharla still couldn't work because I couldn't take care of the kids with my back and all, so we were really in a mess. We got evicted from the apartment and didn't really have anywhere to go. We stayed with Sharla's mom for a while, but there wasn't room in her apartment for the six of us plus her and her new husband. And all of my folks are back east, and they wouldn't have had room for us either.

So, we ended up in a shelter. I can't tell you how that made me feel. A man should be able to take care of his family, and I was a failure. I was as down as I could be and I wallowed in it for quite a while. When I finally came up for air, I looked around to see what I could do for my family to get us out of the mess we were in. I realized that, in some ways, even then, we were lucky. We had each other, and Sharla and I knew we would stick together through thick and thin. And we'd been lucky enough to land in a great shelter—one where we could all stay together and where there were programs to help us get back on our feet.

I won't go through all the details of what happened after that. It's a long story. But basically, Ms. Rafael at the shelter pointed us in some good directions to get help. We talked to a legal aid attorney about how to deal with all of our debts. We got some government subsidies at first, but Ms. Rafael also helped me find a job placement in light industrial where I could work without straining my back. And then we moved into a transitional housing program where we had a small apartment. And now it looks like we're going to get into a rent-controlled house through a program here in town. Ms. Rafael helped us figure out the state health care program so we could get the kids shots and stuff, and Sharla is looking into taking in a couple of extra kids every day to make some money babysitting.

So things are looking up. But once you've gone through something like that, you realize how close you are to the edge all the time. They talk about being "one paycheck away" from homelessness, and that's really true. Because we've always needed every penny to pay the rent and keep food on the table. When I hurt my back and lost that paycheck, we all learned what it was like to fall over the edge. It's an experience I wouldn't wish on anyone, I'll tell you that.

CONCLUSION

Though none of the stories recounted here come from the direct voices of actual individuals, these narratives reflect the nature of homelessness in today's America (see Miller, 1996). First, the voices recount the variety of ways people end up on the streets. Harold had a lifelong struggle with mental illness. Julie had an abusive father and a quick trip into prostitution. Zeke has been "down on his luck" so long he barely remembers another life. These stories all indicate that there is no single "typical" cause for homelessness. Similarly, the voices of those surrounding the homeless express a cacophony of attitudes. Sylvia tries to turn her head and pretend that the street people aren't there, and Paul is tempted to sweep them away so they aren't an eyesore for the tourist trade. In contrast, Father Tim and GeriAnne have devoted their careers to helping those who are homeless, though they find a multitude of frustrations await them in their work. And Maria has developed an intense awareness of the luck and grace of her own life by spending a few afternoons a week helping at a soup kitchen.

None of the narratives in this case present the "true" story of homelessness. Though we may find Meghan's fear of telling her friends that she lives in a shelter heart-wrenching and we may be inspired by Neal's struggle to get his family off the street, these stories only tell a part of the story.

The portion of the story told by Paul, trying to protect his business from urban blight, or Zeke, dumpster diving by day and drinking by night, are equally revealing. Thus, the lesson we learn from these voices is that the "true" story of homelessness is a patchwork of sad, angry, frustrated, and sometimes uplifting tales.

It is only by confronting the complexity of homelessness that we can hope to understand—and perhaps transform—the lives of people on the street. This complexity begins with merely accounting for the homeless—as Barak (1991) noted, estimates of the homeless in America range from 300,000 to 3 million. The complexity of the problem is compounded when one considers the myriad paths that lead to the street and the fragmented programs currently available to serve the homeless. Thus, policymakers and service providers who make simplistic or stereotypic assumptions about homeless individuals will ultimately fail in their quest to "solve" the problem. As proponents of systems theory (e.g., Katz & Kahn, 1978) have taught us for years, the complexity of a system must match the complexity of environmental exigencies it encounters. Thus, our initial goal should be to enhance our understanding of the complicated world in which the homeless live. And perhaps the best first step for understanding is to begin listening to a multitude of voices.

RELEVANT CONCEPTS

coping mechanisms
different perspectives
environmental exigencies
homeless shelters
homelessness
individual impact(s)
societal impacts(s)

DISCUSSION QUESTIONS

1. This case has presented a variety of perspectives on homelessness in the United States today. Which of these stories surprised you the most? Which of these stories most closely matched your preconceptions of homelessness?

2. How would you characterize the various stances taken by domiciled individuals toward the homeless? Which of these stances do you think most closely matches your own? In what ways do these various stances influence homeless individuals and influence local community members?

3. Given what you've learned from these stories, what do you believe are the most important needs that must be met for the homeless? Do you think existing services are capable of providing for the needs of the homeless? Are we doing "too much" for some people?

4. What are the challenges and stressors associated with dealing with the homeless population? What strategies would you suggest for dealing with those stressors?

REFERENCES/SUGGESTED READINGS

Barak, G. (1991). *Gimme shelter: A social history of homelessness in contemporary America.* New York: Praeger.

Jencks, C. (1994). *The homeless.* Cambridge, MA: Harvard University Press.

Katz, D., & Kahn, R. L. (1978). *The social psychology of organizations* (2nd ed.). New York: Wiley.

Liebow, E. (1993). *Tell them who I am: The lives of homeless women.* New York: The Free Press.

Miller, K. (1996). *Gimme shelter: The communication of America's homeless.* In E. B. Ray (Ed.), Communication and disenfranchisement: Social health issues and implications. Mahwah, NJ: Lawrence Erlbaum Associates.

Robertson, M. J., & Greenblatt, M. (Eds.). (1992). *Homelessness: A national perspective.* New York: Plenum.

Snow, D. A., & Anderson, L. (1993). *Down on their luck: A study of homeless street people.* Berkeley: University of California Press.

Walsh, M. E. (1992). *Moving to nowhere: Children's stories of homelessness.* New York: Auburn House.

3 From Pedagogy to Praxis: Affecting Communication in an Inner-City AIDS Clinic

John Kahler
Cook County Hospital and Humana Health Care Plans, Chicago

Barbara F. Sharf
University of Illinois at Chicago

> *Epidemics of particularly dreaded illnesses always provoke an outcry against leniency or tolerance—now identified as laxity, weakness, disorder, corruption: unhealthiness.*
>
> —Sontag (1990, p. 168)

The young girl-woman sits patiently with the 30 other women and various age children waiting to be seen. The waiting room is old; actually it is in the oldest part of the 100-plus-year-old hospital. This is where the Women & Children's Program is housed and is called the HRD Clinic although almost no one other than the clinic personnel know that HRD stands for "human retroviral disease," the causative agent for HIV/AIDS. It was named the HRD Clinic so that both those who are treated here, as well as those who work at the clinic, would not feel "stigmatized." After a 2-hour wait, she is called to the small examining room. Her physician for the morning is a second-year resident who is rotating through the clinic. He is a White man who grew up and was educated in Evanston, an affluent suburb of Chicago. After reviewing her chart, he asks her how she is feeling and whether she is taking all of her medicine. Four medications had been ordered after a recent hospitalization for pneumonia. Although two of the drugs make her sick to her stomach, she has been trying to take them regularly. A quick examination and the 20-minute visit is over. The attending physician comes in and cheerfully inquires how she is feeling. The senior doctor quizzes the junior doctor on some of the specifics of the patient's case: blood count, T-cell level, current medications, and complications of AIDS. At no time does either the senior or the junior physician ask about the current living arrangements of this child nor do they find out her current understanding of the illness and how it might be affecting her life, not simply her physical health. The doctors walk out of the room and tell the frightened, sick young woman that they will see her in 4 weeks and that "everything looks great."

Although the treatment of the aforementioned patient seems to be relatively harsh, in traditional medical education this interaction would be rated favorably. The resident did a complete job of reviewing any interim medical problems with the patient. He performed a physical examination and assessed the complicated laboratory data, as well as medication history and status. In addition, a senior physician supervised his work and even talked with the patient for a brief period. What is missing in this interview is any evidence that the physician either understood or cared for the context of this illness; in other words, how this patient at this time and place was dealing with her illness.

In this chapter we review a model developed to teach elements of the patient–doctor interaction, from a systems theory perspective. In addition, we introduce the *family genogram* as an expansion of this model, which facilitates an individual physician's implementation of systemic concepts into daily work. We use a case drawn from an AIDS clinic to illustrate these concepts in action. The genogram has been advocated in the past (Crouch, 1987) as a means both to integrate data on the physical and mental aspects of health and illness, as well as to graphically display multigenerational patterns of illness and dysfunction. In addition to these functions, we propose that the process of eliciting genogram information can enable practitioners to perceive assumptions embedded within their relationships with patients and their families.

A CROSS-CULTURAL PERSPECTIVE ON MEDICAL ENCOUNTERS

The need for a conceptual model dealing with the many interacting factors affecting the patient–doctor relationship developed from the authors' experiences teaching primary care[1] resident physicians about patient–doctor

[1]Throughout this chapter we use the concept of *primary care* in the context of routine medical care and the patient–doctor interaction. Two major goals of the health care system are: first, to optimize the health of the individual, and second, to provide equity in the distribution of health care resources (Starfield, 1992). As became obvious during the health care reform debates of the early 1990s, these two goals compete for a limited amount of money. *Primary care* is one means by which these two goals—optimization of health and

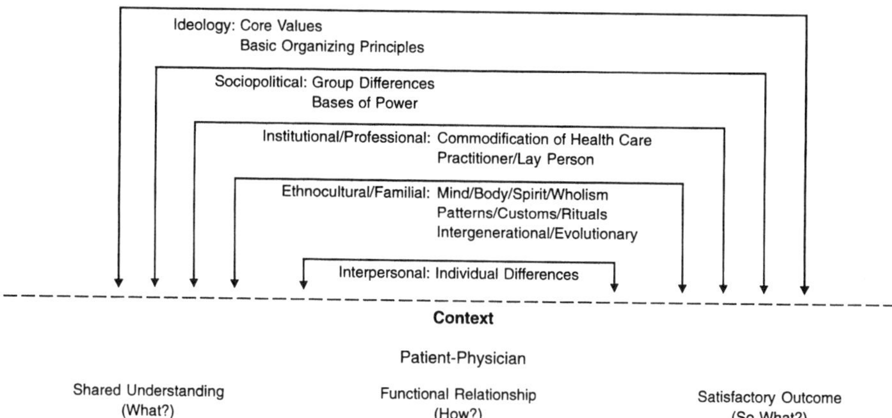

FIG. 3.1. Culturally Sensitive Model of Patient–Physician Communication.

interaction in the Department of Family Practice at the Cook County Hospital in Chicago. We have seen numerous examples of disorganized and even dysfunctional interactions resulting from noncontexualized history gathering. In an attempt to teach about the differing frames of reference, both subtle and overt, that are fundamental to problems arising within medical encounters, we have developed the Culturally Sensitive Model of Patient–Physician Communication (hereafter referred to as CSM; Sharf & Kahler, 1996). This model positions the interpersonal relationship of the individual patient–doctor dyad within a much broader context that includes such differences as race, gender, ethnicity, socioeconomic status, education, cultural beliefs, and family, community, and professional values (see Fig. 3.1).

In practice, each time a physician and patient sit down to discuss the patient's presenting concerns, they bring to that conversation assumptions about the other and the world from sources far removed from the immediate medical context. In order to identify the multiple layers of meanings that may inform a given transaction, our model uses a systems approach of ascending complexity.

---

equity in distributing resources—are balanced. Primary care is an organizational approach that emphasizes the relationship between a patient and a specially trained health care provider (e.g., family practitioner, pediatrician, nurse practitioner). These practitioners address the most common problems in the community by providing preventive, curative, and rehabilitative services to maximize health and well-being to their patient populations. It is care that organizes and rationalizes the deployment of all resources, basic as well as specialized, directed at promoting, maintaining, and improving health. The undergirding to this approach is the ongoing relationship developed between a primary-care provider with his or her patient over time: This is called continuity of care.

At the *interpersonal level,* which is most accessible to change and possible improvement, meaning emanates from the styles and sensibilities of the individual participants, and the resulting quality of rapport and intimate exchange. Interpersonal connotations are always operative but may be superseded by meanings generated at other levels. For example, from the *ethnocultural/familial level* come culturally derived explanations of illness that vary in their inclusion of mind, body, and spirit as well as elements of biomedicine, folk beliefs, and alternative health practices. At the *institutional/professional level,* understandings of health and illness are embedded within and among organizational contexts and distinctions between the perspectives of patients and professionals. The *sociopolitical level* brings to bear the comparative values expressed in social power structures that privilege some demographic groups while marginalizing others. At the most abstract level of complexity is the *ideological level,* the source of basic organizing tenets of a particular social philosophy and core beliefs undergirding national identity. Table 3.1 provides an illustration of how physician and patient assumptions at each level of the model may differ significantly. These are differences we have observed repeatedly within the clinical settings in which we teach.

As a way of teaching physicians-in-training about their own communication with patients, the CSM illustrates how several layers of meaning can be operational simultaneously, that one or more of these layers may predominate, and that the layer(s) of meaning most salient for one person may not be the same for the other. Discussions of particular patient encounters are assessed with the residents in terms of three basic criteria: shared understanding, functionality of relationship, and health care outcomes (Sharf et al., 1991). Nonetheless, moving between this conceptual model and actual behaviors in clinical situations may prove difficult for many trainees.

FROM PEDAGOGY TO PRACTICE

Jim Abbott is a 27-year-old man who has a birth defect that has caused his left arm to be "withered." If you were to see him standing at a major league baseball park, you would think he was like any other fan at the game. But Jim is a pitcher for the Chicago White Sox. Only after watching Jim function can you see the beauty in what seems to be simply a diseased anatomy.

All medical students learn early in school the differences between anatomy and physiology. Think of the concepts of structure and function. Anatomy refers to the *structural* components of the matter at hand, for example, the brain. Physiology refers to the *functional* aspects of the matter,

TABLE 3.1
Systemic Assumptions Affecting Patient–Physician Communication

Levels of Meaning	*Patient*	*Physician*
Interpersonal	Whether voiced or not, patients make their own choices regarding their bodies.	It's important for physicians to control, or at least have a significant role in, medical management.
Ethnocultural/Familial	Doctors may know the best prescription medicines to take, but other people can advise sick people on other ways to feel better.	Home remedies are often dangerous. Even if they do no harm, they have no scientific basis.
Institutional/Professional	Poor people should be suspect of medical research because too often they have been used as guinea pigs.	Medical research is good and necessary. It expands clinical knowledge and improves patient care.
Sociopolitical	Patients with limited education and/or English speaking skills don't want to appear stupid or waste the doctor's time, so many don't ask a lot of questions. Even so, they would like to know what's wrong and how it can be fixed.	The more questions patients ask, the more they wish to know about their condition.
Ideological	In some cultures, communal or family interests take precedence over the interests of an individual.	The individual interests of patients supersede those of families or related communities.

for example, neurotransmission. The two constructs are interdependent, but examining them reveals radically different information. An anatomical analysis shows the skeletal underpinnings, the most gross organization of the process. A physiological analysis reveals a more complex system that is able to individualize function to fit a changing set of variables. Most medical students do quite well in anatomy. Mastery of this discipline involves techniques that the students have used throughout their careers. However, many students start to have problems when they take their first physiology class. The skills here are those of conceptualization and integration of mutually interacting systems. Establishing a relationship and communicating with patients over time calls upon the individual physician to integrate complex interacting systems and is a skill that may be learned only after time and practice. As a means of organizing a complex array of information affecting the patient–physician interaction, the CSM has been quite useful in our attempt to teach the "anatomy" of the interaction. In other words, as a mechanism to teach concepts to groups of students or even to organize a case review with an individual student or resident, the model works well. However, the ultimate purpose of our teaching is to train physicians to be better communicators and to improve their skills at developing meaningful relationships with their patients. The very essence of a "relationship" is the behavioral interaction of the parties involved. This behavior involves developing skills more akin to a "physiological" approach to the relationship. In order to facilitate this transition of content to process, we have now incorporated the use of the family genogram into the clinical application of the model.

The genogram was originally introduced as a means of displaying information about the way genetic diseases were transmitted. A simple example of this is the transmission of sickle cell anemia (see Fig. 3.2). Over the past 10 years, teachers of primary care medicine have attempted to expand the use of the genogram to illustrate the occurrence of dysfunctional patterns such as alcoholism and domestic violence over two or three successive generations. We are now proposing that the family genogram be used as a clinical tool to permit the gathering and organization of intimate, potentially sensitive, multigenerational information. We feel it serves both form and function. Graphically, it permits a physician to obtain and chart family-based information in a precise manner. It also is a technique that enables physicians to feel comfortable in inquiring and detailing information about the unique world that her patient inhabits. When the clinician assesses the information obtained from the family genogram about the individual family, combines this with her knowledge of various sociocultural customs

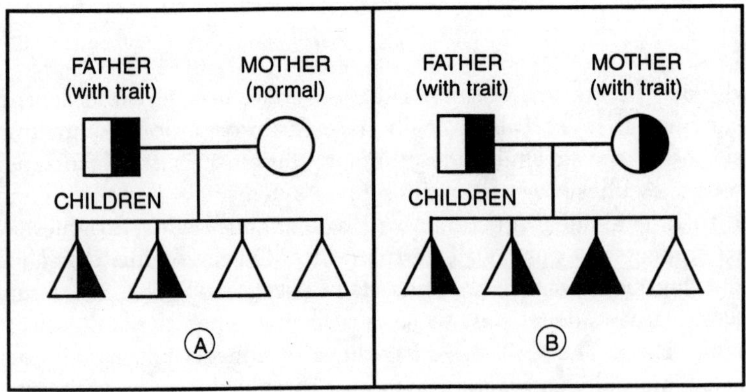

FIG. 3.2. Genogram showing sickle cell inheritance.

and norms, and places these squarely within the framework of the family's socioeconomic conditions, she is operationalizing the culturally sensitive approach to the patient–doctor interaction.

THE WOMEN AND CHILDREN'S PROGRAM

As an example of the organizing power of the family genogram and its use by a physician in her daily work, let us look at the Moynihan family. This family is being followed at the Women & Children's Program at Cook County Hospital, Chicago, a center for the care of HIV-positive women and their children. "The County" is the venue at which large numbers of the medically indigent receive their care. It is the hospital of last resort for large numbers of patients.

Let us begin by drawing the societal frame around the individual patient–doctor interaction. For the most part, it is composed of assumptions about a particular family generated from the larger sociocultural assumptions about those families that appear to be like that one. First, consider the ideological level: Liberal protestations to the contrary, industrialized democracies, be they established or emerging, equate wealth with worth. The patients and their families that come to The County are at the lowest end of any socioeconomic scale. In addition to this, one of the foundation myths of U.S. society is that of personal responsibility and the success of the individual against the collective: the bootstrap metaphor. Most of the patients at the HRD clinic contracted their disease by behaviors that mainstream society deems at least illegal and usually immoral, for example, promiscuous unsafe sexual behavior, often with intravenous drugs. These patients are "responsible" for their disease. This assumption is reinforced if we look at the sociopolitical level. Because these patients are at the lowest level of the socioeconomic ladder, the cost of their care is borne by various governmental bodies; they are at The County being seen at a clinic funded by a federal grant, utilizing a state Medicaid card to receive their medicines. As such, the long-term funding for their care is nonexistent. Whenever public officials need to save money, the first place they turn to is the health benefits of these needy families.

Third are assumptions at the institutional/professional level: Charity care is considered to be "take what you get" care, or "it's better than nothing" care, or, finally, "beggars can't be choosers" care. These patients are disempowered with regard to the choices of health care providers open to them. In previous work, we have referred to this group as disempowered but not disenfranchised (Sharf & Kahler, 1996) in an effort to show that even though resources are available, choices are limited, often lacking any satisfactory options. At teaching hospitals, which are major sites for the provision of care to the medically indigent, most primary care is given by inexperienced clinicians. Remember the young woman in the introduction. The supervision done by the attending (i.e., experienced) physician was more concerned with evaluating the resident's performance than with the quality of care the patient actually received. Although training institutions often consider the former to be a surrogate for the latter, we can easily see that for any individual patient this may not necessarily be so.

This description represents at least part of the context in which the patient–doctor interaction takes place. The assumptions are operative de facto. This negative orientation may be offset by powerful positive forces that will only surface as the clinician struggles to understand the idiosyncracies of each family.

THE MOYNIHAN FAMILY

I first met the Moynihans[2] (see Fig. 3.3) in 1993 when I began caring for Chris. At the time, he was 4 years old and HIV positive. He showed no evidence of his infection and was enrolled in a federally funded research protocol dealing with the natural history of HIV infections and the effects of various medications. The research protocol mandated him to come into the clinic every 4 weeks.[3] During the first few visits, Chris was very reluctant to interact with me. Because he was asymptomatic, the visits would usually take no more than 10 minutes. At the end of each visit I found myself feeling anxious and not at all comfortable with the interaction I had with his aunt, Cecelia. Although all the paperwork was completed and the lab work dutifully ordered, something just was not right. A more junior clinician might blame the hectic nature of the clinic for this feeling of unease. There were always 30 or more patients to be seen and only three small rooms in which to see them. People would come in and go out and there was not even a semblance of privacy. I am sure that this contributed to my discomfort, but I realized that most of this feeling was because I really did not know Chris and his family. I knew his HIV status. I knew his latest blood count and CD4 count, but I did not know him.

At the next visit, I asked Cecelia if she would mind accompanying me with Chris to another area of the Fantus Clinic.[4] We went to my office in

---

[2]The description of the Moynihan family comes from the pediatric practice of the first author, John Kahler, M.D. Therefore, the pronouns "I" and "me" refer to Dr. Kahler. The names of all patients and family members have been changed to maintain their anonymity.

[3]In my private practice, I would have seen Chris much less frequently—no more than every 3 months. Although the increased frequency of visits was not needed from a strictly medical standpoint, it did offer me improved access to this child's narrative.

[4]This is the major outpatient facility for the Cook County Hospital. Over 500,000 visits are made each year to this facility.

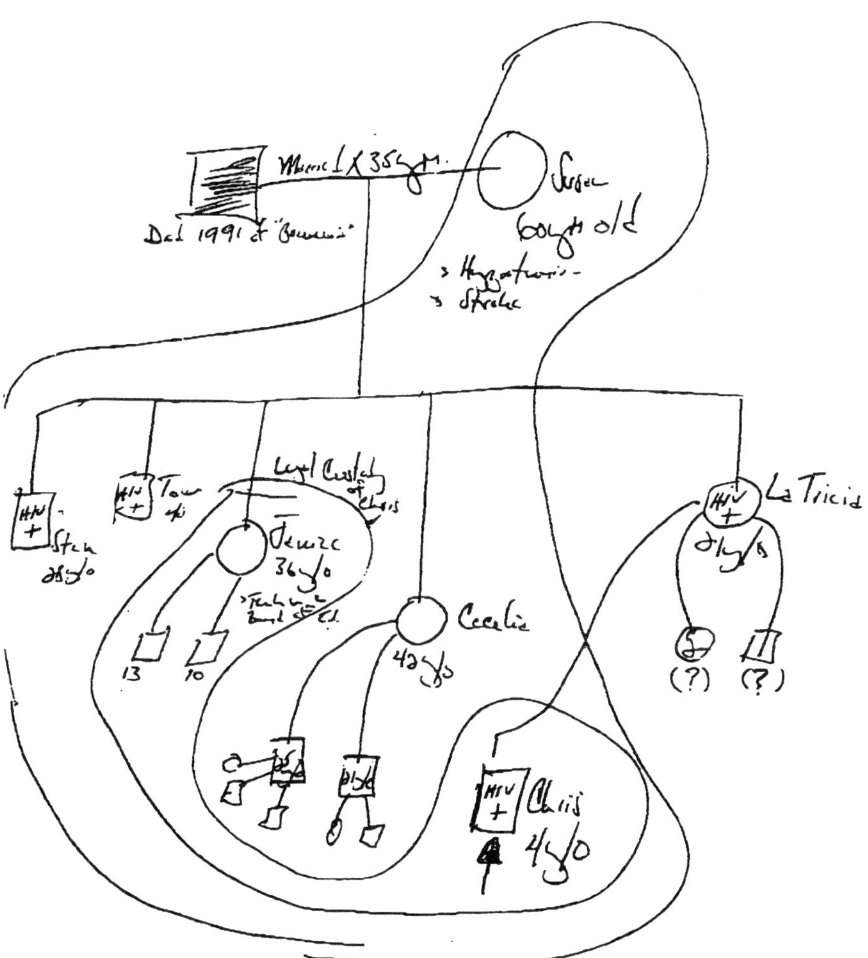

FIG. 3.3. Dr. Kahler's genogram of the Moynihan family. This is a reproduction of the way this material would appear in the medical chart. It has all the flaws and quirks of an individual physician's notations.

the Department of Family Practice. It is quiet, clean, and fairly spacious. I told her that I was sorry I had not taken the time to get to know her before now. I wanted to talk with her in order to get some understanding of how Chris' illness was affecting his family. Even though I have heard similar comments many times, Cecelia's response to me was moving: "Dr. Kahler, I have seen a lot of doctors both for myself as well as for Chris, but no one has ever asked me to tell them about what is going on at home."

Chris is the biological child born to LaTricia, who at this point was a 21-year-old, HIV-positive woman, living on the streets with her two other children, ages 2 and 1, whose HIV status was unknown. LaTricia was described to me as "wasting away to nothing." The only adult I have ever met in this family is Cecelia. At the time I began seeing them, she was 42 years old, an unemployed factory worker and uninfected with HIV. Chris' legal guardian is his 36-year-old aunt, Janice, the only employed member of the Moynihan household family.[5] She is a schoolteacher in the Chicago public schools. She has two biological children, ages 6 and 8, who live in the house also. Cecelia stated to me:

> I don't know what happened. We used to all work. My father worked for 21 years at the post office. My mother had been employed by a small factory which moved to the suburbs. She could have stayed working but it would have taken 2 hours to get to work. My mother sometimes says she doesn't understand what happened to us. She says, "You kids was raised better."

Although Janice does not accompany Chris to his clinic visits, her consent is needed prior to any change in treatment planning for Chris. She is uninfected and reportedly not at high risk for HIV infection. In addition to the three sisters, there initially were two brothers, Stan (28 years old) and Tom (40 years old) who were both HIV positive and living at home. Home is the house of Chris' grandmother, 62-year-old Susan, who has been followed at the Fantus Clinic for the past 20 years. She suffers from diabetes and hypertension. Her only current source of income is disability through Social Security. Susan's husband (Chris' grandfather) died 2 years ago. He had been followed at The County for many years for hypertension and the complications of a stroke that he suffered 5 years before his death. He died at The County during a hospitalization for a relatively minor illness. Cecelia said that the entire family was surprised when her father died. She did not know the name of his doctor because he had been followed for more than 30 years and the doctors "keep coming and going." Cecelia told me that "when Chris was first diagnosed as having AIDS, we talked about not taking him to The County, with Daddy dying there and us not finding out why. I argued that they have the best doctors there." With that, she smiled and looked away from me.

In addition to Chris, there are at least six other children living in the household. They are the products of various relationships between the brothers and women who have "given" the children to Susan "to care for."

[5]In a family genogram, the household family is distinct from the biological family of origin or the nuclear family, which is composed only of those people with whom the child lives. The household family involves all those people of significance who come and go in a child's immediate environment. It is much closer to the concept of extended family.

Most of these relationships are not sanctioned by law and I am unclear as to how these children are supported.

The entire visit took no more than 30 minutes. I did not examine Chris, but told Cecelia that I would look at him again during the next visit in 4 weeks. After gathering this information, I felt much calmer. I finally had a handle on Chris within his family. I knew that the family was attempting to cope with their economic troubles and that Cecelia was assuming the role of Chris' primary caretaker. Over the past 3 years, Chris' health has remained good, but his uncle Tom died from an overdose of heroin. Cecelia and I have developed a close relationship. Recently she shared with me the following information:

> You know Dr. Kahler, I haven't been honest with you. At least, not completely honest. I found out from my doctor that I have HIV. I was ashamed to admit it to you. I honestly haven't been doing anything for quite a while, but I had been involved with a lot of drugs earlier in my life. I try to figure out why, but I guess I was just depressed. Each time I come to the office, you try to cheer me up about Chris and I felt that I wanted you to know about me too.

ANATOMY AND PHYSIOLOGY, REDUX

Look again at the Moynihan family genogram. The graphic representation of the household family leads to an impression of chaos and disorganization. There are numerous children from several unsustained relationships all living under one roof without their biological mother or any semblance of a responsible man. Only one adult is employed. Dependency, disease, and dysfunction appear to dominate the family structure. However, there are other perspectives that one comes away with during the process of sketching the genogram, attitudes and details that do not lend themselves to graphic representation. In fact, Cecelia talks both hopefully and realistically: "Let me tell you, Dr. Kahler, since Chris has stayed healthy for all these years, I think (and I pray) that he might be one of those children you hear about who beat this disease." At another time, she said, "Our family is comfortable that Chris is in good hands at this time and if he gets sicker, you will be able to help him not hurt." Where one might posit dependency, Cecelia talks about the strengths of the family:

> Janice and me are working together for the first time in our life. When I was younger I didn't understand the importance of my family. We are trying as hard as we can to let Mama know we appreciate all she tried to do for us. I know that I have disappointed her by all that I've done in my life, but I'm going to try and make it up over these next few years.

In other words, the richness of this story can only be filled in from the narrative of the interview.

When a health care provider enters the affective domain with her patient, it can be scary, but it is always rewarding. The process of eliciting the family genogram changed and deepened the relationship between Dr. Kahler and Cecelia (and, by extension, her family), by allowing him to express interest and increase understanding. It also permitted Cecelia to unburden herself of some of the shame and blame that accompanies all chronic illness, but is supercharged with an illness that carries all the negative connotations as AIDS.

As we stated at the outset, the Culturally Sensitive Model is a conceptual-cognitive way of orienting doctors-in-training to the complex systems that influence their interactions with patients. As an extension of this approach, the family genogram becomes a tool by which health care providers can elicit information that will help them broaden their understanding of their patient families. The conversations that take place in relation to the genogram permit the richness of the individual family's coping styles to come to the fore. In addition, the family genogram is a powerful technique by which we as teachers can help our students begin to understand the importance of the narratives of patients and their families to their daily clinical work. In the words of physicist and Nobel laureate Victor Weisskopf (as quoted in Kabat-Zinn, 1994):

> It was a great pleasure to observe with my own eyes and with utmost clarity all the details I had only seen on photographs before. As I looked at all that, I realized that the room had begun to fill with people, and one by one they too peeked into the telescope. I was told that those were astronomers attached to the observatory, but they had never before had the opportunity of looking directly at the objects of their investigations. I can only hope that this encounter made them realize the importance of such direct contacts. (pp. 186–187)

RELEVANT CONCEPTS

affective domain
anatomy and physiology/structure and function
context of illness
conversational process
Culturally Sensitive Model
family genogram
physician and patient assumptions
primary care
systems perspective

DISCUSSION QUESTIONS

1. Why is it important to think about patient-physician communication in relation to a multilayered system of meanings? Is the model presented here, in fact, "culturally sensitive"? Why or why not?

2. What are some reasons that doctors may have trouble translating the concepts represented in the Culturally Sensitive Model into actual communicative behaviors during their interviews with patients?

3. Explain the difference between anatomy and physiology. How well does this metaphor work as a way of describing communication? Is it applicable to other than a health care setting?

4. What were your initial assumptions when you looked at the genogram and read the overall description of the Moynihan family? Did these ideas change at all after you read about Cecelia's conversation with Dr. Kahler? If so, in what ways?

5. What assumptions might a practitioner make about you and your family based on a pictorial genogram? How might these assumptions change if you were given an opportunity to describe and explain your family's situation?

6. What are some of the assumptions you have made about health care practitioners that you have seen? On what were these assumptions based?

REFERENCES/SUGGESTED READINGS

Abraham, L. K. (1993). *Mama might be better off dead: The failure of health care in urban America*. Chicago: University of Chicago Press.

Crouch, M. A. (1987). Using the genogram (family tree) clinically. In M. A. Crouch & L. Roberts (Eds.), *The family in medical practice: A family systems primer* (pp. 174–192). New York: Springer-Verlag.

Kabat-Zinn, J. (1994). *Wherever you go, there you are: Mindfulness meditation in everyday life*. New York: Hyperion.

Sharf, B. F., Kahler, J., Foley, R. P., Grant, D., Bomgaars, M., & Harper, S. (1991). *A shared understanding: Bridging racial and socioeconomic differences in doctor-patient communication* (instructor's manual). Chapel Hill, NC: Health Sciences Consortium.

Sharf, B. F., & Kahler, J. (1996). Victims of the franchise: A culturally sensitive model of teaching patient–doctor communication in the inner city. In E. B. Ray (Ed.), *Communication and disenfranchisement: Social health issues and implications*. Mahwah, NJ: Lawrence Erlbaum Associates.

Sontag, S. (1990). *Illness as metaphor and AIDS and its metaphors*. New York: Anchor Books.

Starfield, B. (1992). *Primary care: Concept, evaluation, and policy*. New York: Oxford University Press.

4 *"I Just Can't Afford It": Overcoming Barriers Facing Women Living in Poverty*

Alicia A. Marshall
Texas A&M University

Janet K. McKeon
Michigan State University

FACING THE REALITY

"I just can't afford to get it checked," Ruby said with a hint of frustration in her voice. Ruby's coworkers in the kitchen weren't sure if she was trying to convince them or to convince herself. None were convinced, especially Ruby. Ruby Green was a 46-year-old widow, mother of six, and grandmother of two. She worked hard as a cook and dishwasher at the neighborhood grade school. She was there every Monday through Friday. Her coworkers couldn't remember a day when she had called in sick. She was just always there. She never complained about the minimum wages or the hot conditions of the kitchen or the back-breaking work of standing over the stove or sink 8 hours a day. And she hadn't even mentioned this, until now.

Ruby was a proud woman; everyone knew that and respected her for it. Supporting herself and her kids was tough to do on her limited wages. She couldn't afford any insurance; it was hard enough to keep food on the table and clothes on their backs. She refused to take any charity or help from friends. She hated using the food stamps for which she qualified, but she did. She never did anything for herself. Her kids and grandchildren were her top priority; their needs always came first.

Rose, her oldest, had two children, Tommy (5 years old) and Dottie (2 years old). The three of them lived with Ruby and four of Rose's siblings so that the little ones could be taken care of while Rose worked as a beautician's assistant at a local salon. Ruby's son Dick was a mechanic and lived on his own in a nearby town. John, her next boy, was 20 years old now and was working part time to pay for night classes at the community college. He still lived at home. Ruby was so proud of him. Then there was Sally, 15 years old and growing up quicker than Ruby could imagine. And finally there was Annie (9 years old) and Billy (now 6). Annie was becoming a big help around the house, taking care of Tommy and Dottie after school and helping Sally with the cleaning and the cooking. Ruby was proud of all her children. She had raised them to work hard and to take care of one another because "no one else would," as she told them often.

Ruby had married her high school sweetheart, Jack. After high school Jack had become a construction worker. They had lived in a little house in the same neighborhood where they had grown up. All those years since high school Ruby had stayed home to raise their children. But there had been an accident and Jack was gone now, and Ruby had had to find a job with only a high school education and limited vocational skills. It had been tough, but she had finally found her job at the school. She loved the children and they loved her. "Mamma Ruby" they called her. She was always after them to finish their food, especially their vegetables, as if they were all her own children. Her coworkers loved her too. She was the best listener around, always willing to give advice, or a shoulder to cry on, or just a big hug. She was always telling everyone that they had to look out for each other, they were like family, and nothing's more important than that.

It was while cleaning the kitchen after lunch one day that Ruby had casually mentioned to her coworkers that she had "found something." "A lump I guess. Won't go away, but I'm sure it's nothing. And anyway, I just can't afford to have it checked." It had all started close to 6 weeks ago now when Ruby had first found the lump in her breast while taking a shower. She never did those self-exams that she'd heard about for years; she didn't know how to do them right and assumed she wouldn't find anything anyway. But there it was; a lump the size of one of her grandson's marbles.

Of course her first response was, "It's nothing. I'm just getting old and lumpy." But it kept creeping back into her mind day after day, and it didn't seem to be going away. "Look," she told herself, "it's nothing. And if it is something, there's nothing I can do about it anyway. Getting sick is just the luck of the draw." She couldn't bring herself to consider the possibility of cancer; she couldn't even think the word. Everyone knew getting cancer was a death sentence. You get cancer and you die. It was happening all around her it seemed these days. And what about the children? She couldn't leave them. Who would pay the heating bills and buy the food? She took comfort in the fact that no one else in her family had had cancer. She thought that was a good sign and that she wasn't likely to get it, but she really wasn't sure.

To tell the truth, she really didn't know much about cancer, like where it came from, for example. But then again, it didn't seem like anyone else knew either. She'd gotten sick and tired of hearing all the warnings about this causing cancer or that causing cancer. She had finally just tuned it all out. Those overpaid experts couldn't agree with one another on who should even be worried. Some said women over 40 years old, others said over 50. Well, she had to worry about putting food on the table every night. Those people couldn't relate to what she was going through. She had seen a commercial the other night on TV where the governor was sitting in his plush living room talking about how important it was that women got some type of test for breast cancer. It was easy for him to say; he could afford to pay for his wife to get the test. What did he know about what Ruby and her friends went through day to day just to survive? And what good would a test do? If she had it she had it. Why find out that you're dying?

Ruby finally decided to mention it to her friends at work. Maybe then she would stop thinking about it. She was closest to Harriet and Doris. They had been working in the kitchen as long as Ruby. They were both like sisters to her. When Ruby mentioned the lump, Harriet and Doris both took it in stride. They told her not to worry, it was probably nothing. They were calm, but they wouldn't let Ruby ignore it any longer. Doris had lost another friend to breast cancer a few years ago and she wasn't going to let Ruby just stand by passively not knowing and not giving herself a fighting chance if it did turn out to be cancer. Unlike most of the women she knew, Doris believed that people did have some control over their own lives and bodies and that determination and fight went a long way to overcoming some pretty bad things that could come along.

LOOKING FOR ANSWERS

The first thing they had to do was to find out more about what Ruby should do. The best sources they knew were their friends and family members. Surely someone in their neighborhood knew something about getting tested for breast cancer. Most of the women they talked to had never been tested; it was just too expensive or too complicated. Harriet knew that the test was called a mammogram. When she talked to some of her friends, most of them thought it was some sort of painful procedure that involved clamping your breast into a vice. One thing was for sure, most of the women said they wouldn't want to get the test. "Why tempt fate by looking for something?" one woman stated. "I just plain wouldn't want to know the results, so why have the test in the first place?" questioned another. "My cousin had one of those mammograms done and she said it really hurt. Who wants to go through that?" The concerns went on and on. Many were embarrassed by the whole thing. Several said they just wouldn't be able to take the time off from work and lose the wages. The more women Harriet and Doris talked to the longer the list grew of reasons not to get the screening done. As one woman put it, "There are too many walls to climb over. I just don't have the energy." They were hearing many concerns, but very few answers.

Despite the shared concerns and fears over the screening, the women all acknowledged that breast cancer was a dangerous thing. Most women knew at least one person personally that had struggled with cancer. Harriet and Doris were also struck by the fact that few of their friends, themselves included, knew exactly what a mammogram did, what it would tell them, or why it was so important. They were also collectively unsure as to how to go about getting one, especially given their limited resources.

While Harriet and Doris were on their information-seeking mission, Ruby had decided to confide in Rose, her oldest, and to talk to some of her other women friends to see what they knew. She certainly didn't want to worry anyone, particularly any of the children, but she thought at least Rose should know what was happening. Ruby still wasn't convinced that she should bother finding out what the lump was, or that she would even be able to afford to have any tests done. Nonetheless, Rose convinced her mother to let her at least call around and see about getting her in to see a doctor somewhere. Surely somewhere someone would be able to see her despite having no insurance and limited funds.

Rose was discouraged, to say the least, by what she found. Given they lived in a large urban area, there was a free clinic downtown. Unfortunately, her mother would have to take three different buses to get there, they only saw patients three afternoons a week due to a limited number of willing health care providers, and there was an 8-week waiting list to get an appointment. Even if she could get downtown and get an appointment, the clinic didn't have the mammography equipment; they would have to refer her to one of the area hospitals, which would require insurance.

One day while at work in the beauty salon, one of the customers was talking about a coupon book she had recently received. "I got over $200 dollars worth of coupons free just for going in and having a mammogram done!" the customer exclaimed. This caught Rose's attention immediately. "How did you say you got those coupons?" Rose asked. The customer responded:

> Well, a neighbor of mine had heard about a program down at the public health department that provided mammograms and Pap smears for virtually nothing if you aren't insured or able to afford such tests otherwise. I called up, made an appointment, and when I went in they handed me this coupon book. Here, take one of these coupons for the drugstore on the corner. The

coupon has the program's phone number on it if you want to call. You know, that X ray wasn't as bad as I thought it would be. Call them, honey, you'll feel better.

Rose called the program later that day while on her break. She talked to a very friendly and helpful woman named Laura and found out all about the program that the customer had mentioned. They did in fact provide low-cost or even free breast and cervical cancer screening for women over 40 who were without insurance and/or living on limited resources. Once Rose explained the circumstances Laura assured Rose that her mother would qualify. Laura also told Rose a number of things that she felt would help convince her mother to make an appointment as soon as possible to have her lump checked out. First and foremost, Laura wanted Rose to know that the absolute best defense against breast cancer known at this point is early detection. If cancer is detected early, the probability of survival is very high.

The Breast and Cervical Cancer Control Program (the name of their specific federally funded program) provides both clinical breast exams performed primarily by female health care providers as well as mammograms. In addition, clients are taught how to do monthly self breast exams, the third method recommended to assist in early detection of breast cancer. Laura acknowledged that most women are afraid of mammograms simply because of the unknown. Laura assured Rose that a mammogram is a brief X ray of the breast that may be slightly uncomfortable, but should not be painful for the woman if done properly. The procedure consists of two appointments: The first consists of the clinical breast exam and Pap smear, and the second is for the mammogram. Laura also wanted Rose to know that the program will assist in transportation or child care if that would help. Laura stressed to Rose that even though women may think they are not at risk (e.g., because they haven't had anyone with cancer in their immediate family), just by virtue of being a woman they are at risk and should be screened regularly.

Rose felt relieved by the end of their conversation. There *was* a program out there for women like her mother. Rose had learned quite a bit during her brief conversation with Laura. Knowing how her mother's friends don't trust or pay attention to the media much, she asked Laura if it might be possible for someone to come in person to talk to a group of the women in their neighborhood about the program. Laura happily agreed. One of their primary missions in the program was to conduct educational programs out in the community to increase awareness of the importance of early-detection screening and to motivate women to enroll in their program. They were happy to do anything to better inform the women, calm some of their fears, and motivate them to engage in regular screening so that they wouldn't have to go through what Rose's mother was having to go through. As they were saying goodbye, Laura told Rose to have her mother call if she had any questions and ask for her specifically. She ended by telling Rose to remind her mother that this was a very positive, potentially life-saving thing that she can do for herself, her children, and her grandchildren.

That night Rose asked Harriet and Doris over to their house for coffee so that the four women could share with one another what they had learned. Between them, they had talked to a number of women in their neighborhood. They were struck by how similar the comments were across all the women they had talked to. "You know, one thing that I thought about was the fact that this just isn't something we talk about much. But once I brought up the subject, everyone seemed to want to talk about it and share their stories and concerns with someone else," Harriet observed. "I had that same experience," Doris commented. "I was at a Tupperware party a few nights ago, and once I said something about having a friend who had found a lump and was looking for medical help, we spent the rest of the night talking about what we knew and what we didn't know."

As the women compared "notes" they found quite a lot of consistency in what the neighborhood women really wanted to talk and find out about. It was very clear that they generally wanted to be better educated and have greater access to "just plain information" without all the confusing numbers and disclaimers that seem to be attached to everything these days. Most of the women were confused by what they were hearing on TV or reading in magazines about who was at risk and what they should be doing about it. Rose noticed that it sounded like the women really wanted to know much more about what to do about breast cancer, but at the same time they had an attitude similar to Ruby's that if they got breast cancer there would be nothing they could do about it.

"What do you think the women really want to know specifically?" Rose asked. "Well, a lot of the women I talked to wanted to know once and for all who exactly is at risk for breast cancer and who should be worried?" Harriet said. "Yeah, and they also want to know what to do if they find something like a lump, just like we're trying to find out. I can't tell you how many women asked that I let them know what I find out *if* I find out anything," Doris added.

The biggest issue was cost; the women just saw no way of being able to afford getting tested for cancer. A lot of the women also wanted to know, in basic terms, what kind of tests were done. What exactly is a mammogram? Is it as painful as it sounded? Isn't it dangerous to have regular X rays given the radiation? The women also clearly needed to be convinced that having such a test was useful and important. They still saw little need in finding out that they were dying of breast cancer. Throughout the evening the women put together quite a list of questions the neighborhood women wanted answers to. "I'll tell you one more thing. *Everyone* wanted to talk about the 'change of life.' Guess we should start having 'health talk' parties to get us together to talk about these things!" Harriet added. Rose thought that wasn't such a bad idea. It was clear from their discussion this evening that this was something the women in the neighborhood wanted to do, whether they knew it consciously or not.

At this point Rose began telling her mother and her friends about her conversation with Laura at the health department. Rose reported all that Laura had told her about the screening program that was available. First of all, Rose told the women that they were all at risk of getting breast cancer simply because they were women. The biggest risk factors were family history and age. If your mother or a sister had breast cancer, you were more likely to get it as well. Rose also reported that the probability of getting breast cancer went up significantly after the age of 50. Other factors such as experiencing a first childbirth after the age of 30, or never having children, as well as either beginning menstruation early in life (before age 11) or experiencing late menopause were also considered risk factors. What had surprised Rose though was that nearly 75% of those women diagnosed with breast cancer didn't have any of these risk factors.

"What did she say about diet and stuff?" Harriet asked. Rose remembered Laura saying that researchers were still examining the effect of diet, obesity, alcohol use, and taking an oral contraceptive for several years on breast cancer. The one thing that stuck out in Rose's mind was that all these factors are merely associated with breast cancer, researchers haven't identified conclusively what causes it yet. That means they can't prevent the disease. What can be done is doing everything possible to detect it early so that it can be dealt with aggressively.

Ruby had been quiet most of the evening. Rose had been watching her to see how she was taking all this discussion; it was, after all, because of the lump in her breast that they had started all this information seeking in the first place. "What are you thinking, Mom?" she finally asked.

"I was just wondering if there were any other symptoms that maybe I should look for," Ruby replied. Rose had thought of that same thing when she was talking to Laura. Laura had told her that other warning signs included a change in the shape of the breast, puckering or swelling, pain or tenderness, and discharge. Luckily, Ruby had not experienced any of these other symptoms. "And what exactly would I have to do to get this silly little lump checked out?" she asked. Rose proceeded to tell her all she had learned about what a mammogram was and what exactly she could expect when she made an appointment. Ruby liked that the examiner would be a woman; that would help her feel less embarrassed. A man just wouldn't be able to understand what she was going through or what it felt like. She also was relieved to hear that the procedure shouldn't be as painful as she had feared. Ruby and her friends were most relieved to hear about the minimal cost and the assistance with transportation to the appointment.

"Well," Harriet began, "I don't know about you, but the program sure sounds good to me. I would go in in a minute if I had found that lump. It's probably nothing. But why not go in and have it checked, just for peace of mind if nothing else. You are always doing things for others, why not do something like this for yourself?" "And remember what Rose told us," Doris added, "it sounds like even if it is something, if they catch it early there is something they can do about it."

"You know, you really shouldn't wait until you find a lump to get a mammogram done. Laura said women over the age of 40 should be getting them every year or two," Rose said. "She told me that a mammogram can detect a lump up to 2 years before you or a doctor might be able to feel it." Rose paused, then said, "I have an idea. Why don't the three of you make appointments together? Seems like it might be less scary if you went in together. I'd even go in with you, if you'd like. And don't forget about the coupon book that I told you about that helped us find out about this program in the first place! What do you say?"

After thinking about it briefly, the women agreed there really weren't any good reasons they could think of to not go in for a mammogram. Ruby was relieved that her friends were willing to go in with her. She still was frightened by what she might find out, but at least she knew there was a program set up to help her. Finally they all agreed to call first thing the next morning.

REACHING OUT TO WOMEN LIVING IN POVERTY

The next afternoon at their weekly staff meeting, Laura was recounting her conversation with Rose to everyone. "Did you say the mother's name was Ruby?" asked the receptionist. "She called in this morning and made an appointment and said two of her friends wanted to come in at the same time. Hey, Laura, your talk must have worked!" Laura was relieved that Ruby was coming in and that her time spent with Rose on the phone had brought in three more women for screening. Nevertheless, she was distressed that the women had not heard about the program until recently. Thank goodness for those coupon books; at least they were doing what they had been intended to do and had gotten women started talking.

Over the last 6 months Laura and her staff had tried everything they could think of to reach and motivate the women to enroll in the program. They had placed ads in the local newspapers and in the free *Shoppers Guide.* They had distributed flyers to local businesses like grocery stores, drug stores, bars, and restaurants. They had TV and radio spots running periodically telling the audience about the importance of regular mammograms. They had even gone around and educated store owners in hopes that they would talk it up among their customers. These approaches just weren't working. Only a fraction of the women that qualified were actually enrolling in the program.

The staff members had then started trying more labor intensive but creative approaches to reaching out to the women. It had become clear to Laura that they needed to use more direct contact approaches. That is, the women needed to be contacted face-to-face, and given the opportunity to ask questions and to be convinced in person that the exam was necessary. They started having tables set up at local discount stores where women could stop and ask questions. They went out and talked to community groups, and even talked to small groups of friends that gathered informally wanting to learn more about breast cancer. The times they had spent talking to members of the local foster grandparent program had also seemed to work. They had tried a direct-mailing and phone-calling campaign as well. It had taken a lot of time and energy, but it had resulted in more women coming in to the program.

These direct strategies seemed to work better. When Laura had the opportunity to ask women why they worked, the women reported that they had made the women feel special, like someone cared about them specifically. The other message Laura had heard loud and clear was that word-of-mouth was the best advertisement they could get. Even more powerful was the impact past participants in the program had on potential clients. If a trusted friend said that she had gone in, had a mammogram, and that it was a positive experience, that went a long way to convince the women to come in themselves. The network throughout this community was clearly very strong and powerful. If she and her staff could just figure out how to tap into that network and get the women to encourage one another to come in, then they would be a success. She was sure of it. The challenge they faced now was simply coming up with those outreach strategies. But the effort would be worth it if they could reach this particular group of isolated and disenfranchised women. More than ever Laura was determined to do all she could to increase the number of women having mammograms. It was their best line of defense in the fight against breast cancer.

"OK, everyone. We have a lot of work to do and a lot of women yet to reach . . ."

FACING THE CHALLENGE OF BREAST CANCER

Ruby's doubts, fears, and experiences are common among disenfranchised women living in poverty today. Breast cancer in the United States has reached epic proportions recently, striking an estimated 182,000 women each year (American Cancer Society, 1994). Approximately 90% of women diagnosed with breast cancer when the cancer is still localized reach the critical 5-year survival mark (National Center for Health Statistics, 1991). Unfortunately, women like Ruby living in poverty are less likely to engage in annual check-ups and/or early-detection disease screening. Generally, there is a dramatic underutilization of mammograms among older, poorer, and less educated women (AMC Cancer Research Center, 1992). Less than 22% of women living in poverty and over the age of 40 ever have a mammogram, thus virtually eliminating the chance of early detection and survival for these disenfranchised women (U.S. Dept. of Health and Human Services, 1990).

Fortunately, increasing the use of mammography screening among women living in poverty has become a priority in the United States in recent years. One such effort is the Breast and Cervical Cancer Control Program (BCCCP) sponsored by the Centers for Disease Control and Prevention described earlier. This program, initiated in 1991, was designed to aid low-income and/or uninsured women by providing low-cost or free cancer screenings. The BCCCP, now available in 24 states across the country, provides comprehensive screening for those cancers that are prevalent in women. The standard exam includes a clinical breast exam, Pap smear, pelvic exam, mammogram, and appropriate referral to community providers for follow-up treatment if abnormalities are detected in the screening examinations.

The primary goal of the BCCCP is to reduce the mortality rate in women from breast and cervical cancer by increasing early detection through regular screening. Furthermore, the program has as its goal to educate low-income women about breast and cervical cancer and the vital role regular screening plays in early detection and thus surviving cancer. Each participating state has the freedom to establish the program as it sees fit: Some are run through local health departments as the one described previously; others have established community-based coalitions through private offices and hospitals. Approximately half of the programs are managed through the state's department of public health. Regardless of the model being employed, the program's mission is to inform and motivate disenfranchised women living in poverty in hopes of decreasing the rising rate of cancer deaths facing the members of this population.

The outreach efforts described previously to educate these disenfranchised women about breast health and to motivate them to enroll in the program have been tried in a variety of programs. Sadly, although many programs have experienced some successes with these strategies, overall the number of women actually taking advantage of this program is still less than the total number of women who should be enrolling in the program. More and more programs are calling upon public health communication specialists to design and implement creative outreach strategies that acknowledge the unique circumstances and concerns facing this particular population. The goal of the program, and similar programs established to provide preventive health care measures to the disenfranchised, is still to effectively reach the members of this population and to motivate them to proactively engage in desirable health behaviors. It has become clear with the passage of time that the success of programs such as the one described here rests on the quality of the health communication outreach strategies employed.

Ruby was lucky. Through the efforts of her daughter, she found out about the availability of the screening program and was able to take advantage of it and have her lump diagnosed. She was also lucky in that she was among the approximately 75% of women who develop benign rather than malignant lumps that are not cancerous. Thousands of other women, however, are not so lucky. They continue to be uninformed and virtually unreached regarding health-related opportunities and services designed specifically to meet their needs. Effectively reaching the women of this disenfranchised population will only occur if a strong partnership is forged between health and communication experts.

RELEVANT CONCEPTS

health locus of control
perceived barriers
perceived susceptibility
sources of health-related information

DISCUSSION QUESTIONS

1. Identify some of the barriers that were operating to prevent Ruby and/or her friends and neighbors from having regular breast cancer screening performed. How might these barriers be reduced or eliminated through a public health campaign?

2. Contrast Ruby's, Rose's, and Doris' orientation or philosophy about health and illness (i.e., health locus of control). How might their differing orientations affect their health-related behaviors, such as seeking out health-related information or having regular screenings done?

3. What sources of health-related information were most relied on among the women in the case? What source characteristics were seen as most credible? Not credible?

4. What unique strategies should health communicators try in an attempt to motivate these disenfranchised women to engage in desirable health behaviors such as early-detection cancer screening?

REFERENCES/SUGGESTED READINGS

AMC Cancer Research Center. (1992). *Breast and cervical screening: Barriers and use among specific populations.* Denver: AMC Cancer Research Center.

American Cancer Society. (1989). *Cancer and the poor: A report to the nation.* Atlanta: Author.

American Cancer Society. (1994). *Cancer facts and figures: 1994.* Atlanta: Author.

Bergner, L., & Yerby, A. S. (1968). Low income and barriers to use of health services. *The New England Journal of Medicine, 278,* 541–546.

Childers, T., & Post, J. A. (1975). *The information poor in America.* Metuchen, NJ: Scarecrow Press.

Freimuth, V. S. (1990). The chronically uninformed: Closing the knowledge gap in health. In E. B. Ray & L. Donohew (Eds.), *Communication and health: Systems and applications* (pp. 171–186). Hillsdale, NJ: Lawrence Erlbaum Associates.

National Center for Health Statistics. (1991). *Health, United States, 1991.* Hyattsville, MD: U.S. Department of Health and Human Services.

U.S. Department of Health and Human Services. (1990). *Healthy people 2000: National health promotion and disease prevention objectives.* Washington, DC: U.S. Government Printing Office.

PART II

ISSUES RELATED TO FAMILY

5 *The Baby Shower: Rituals of Public and Private Joy and Sorrow*[1]

Fredi Avalos-C'deBaca
Patricia Geist
Julie L. Gray
Ginger Hill
San Diego State University

Susan and Dave approached the house tentatively. Although they had accepted the shower invitation with enthusiasm, Susan knew that Dave must be feeling as nervous as she was. It was not as though they had not looked forward to this event. It was going to be a reunion of sorts. With so many of their oldest and closest friends scattered across the country, it was rare to have as large and complete a gathering as this promised to be. At the bottom of the invitation, the host had written, "It will be just like old times." Susan thought, maybe that's what we're afraid of, feeling like the old times again.

As Susan and her family approached the brick-lined entryway, she looked through the large plate-glass window and recognized many of the familiar faces she saw inside. She could see that some of them were smiling at her. She looked quickly at Dave and her two daughters and took a deep breath. I have my girls now, everything has changed, she reminded herself. But in spite of her effort to block the emotions, it did begin to feel a little like "old times."

[1]This case study was designed around four extensive interviews with a couple who experienced the pain of infertility. Although the case is set in a hypothetical context, it is an accurate representation of the dilemmas faced by the couple and members of their circle of family and friends.

However, it is important to note that a case study, by definition, is limited in scope. The infertile couple and their friends in this study were predominantly Anglo, upper middle class, and educated. As such, the case offers only a glimpse of the reality experienced by infertile couples belonging to a certain socioeconomic segment of our society.

It really was wonderful to see so many of the familiar faces again. Susan was glad they decided to arrive a little early. They had been at the party for at least an hour without having had a chance to say hello to everyone. But there was time. Susan found herself with a large group of people, being ushered into the newly decorated nursery. Sandy, the mother-to-be, was animated as she detailed the features of a yellow changing table against the wall. She and her husband, Doug, had obviously spent a great deal of time and money to make the baby welcome. Susan's emotions were bittersweet as she watched the excitement in Sandy's face. At least today, I can feel genuinely happy for Sandy; 13 years ago I don't know if that would have been possible, Susan thought to herself. "Susan, can I ask you something?"

Susan smiled warmly at the woman standing next to her. "Of course Mary, what is it?" She was almost glad for the interruption. Susan had met Mary at a birthday party of a mutual friend 2 months earlier. Mary had confided to Susan that she and her husband Frank had recently discovered they were infertile.

Today, Mary had approached Susan almost shyly. "I want to ask you about your girls. I mean, I know that they are adopted."

"I'm always happy to talk about my girls," Susan replied.

"Well, what was it like the first time you saw Cameron?" The question did not surprise Susan. She and Dave had always been open about their infertility and the fact that both their daughters were adopted. She had been asked questions like this since they had made the decision to adopt their first child, Cameron, 8 years before.

"She was a ginger, that's what my husband calls redheads, and I knew from the moment I saw her and held her that I could not imagine feeling more bonded or in love with anyone more than I was with her at that moment."

Susan turned and faced Mary. They looked at each other and Susan could sense the woman's pain. She felt as though she could almost reach out and touch it. Susan and Mary followed a very pregnant Sandy into the living room. Sandy had gained at least 40 pounds.

Susan watched the look on Mary's face. She felt a sudden pang of sadness when she thought that Mary may never know what it would be like to hold a child of her own for the first time. Although Susan and Sandy had arrived at motherhood through different channels, Susan was certain that the feelings she had for Cameron and Ava could not be any different than a birth mother's love for her own children.

Susan and Mary joined a large group of men and women who formed a circle around the expecting couple as they began to tear into the precariously stacked blue and pink boxes at their side. Susan thought, I like this new tradition, men and women coming together to celebrate a new life. It was so different 13 years ago when she and Dave were trying to conceive.

Susan tried not to stare at the sad young woman standing next to her. She understood the well-spring of emotions that must be festering within her. Ten years ago, she herself had been another sad young woman trying desperately to hide her own pain and anger from many of the same faces that stood before them now.

She wanted to put her arm around the woman and tell her that it would be all right but something stopped her. Susan remembered how desperately she wanted her friends to understand. In retrospect, she realized that perhaps she had been a little unfair. How could she have expected anybody who hadn't been through the pain and isolation of infertility to really understand? She cringed when she remembered that she had actually been paranoid enough to believe that some of her friends had been doing things deliberately to hurt her. She thought of her husband Dave's quiet response to her accusations.

"Sometimes I feel the same way too, and then I feel guilty for having those feelings. I mean is it really their fault they started having kids and baby showers? Are they supposed to not be happy because we are having trouble? They have to live their lives too, Susan."

On an intellectual level, Susan could not fault Dave's logic. Of course it was not their fault. But she could still feel the blood rush to her face as she remembered other baby showers; the seemingly endless stream of gifts that were passed from woman to woman and how she struggled to find the words and the voice to express the inane obligatory commentary expected for each one.

"Oh how precious." "That's adorable." "She'll need lots of these."

To Susan the gifts represented someone else's dream, and someone else's child. Each one seemed to stand as a monument to her and her husband's own shattered dreams of parenting a child they conceived.

She felt a little guilty remembering how envious and jealous she had become of people that had children. Even today the memory stings.

I still think they could have been more sensitive to our situation. I don't know. Maybe Dave was right. How could they have understood?

THE FRIENDS

Susan looked around the room. Overall she and Dave had been lucky. With a few exceptions, their circle of friends had remained close and consistent. Susan smiled when she saw Jack, a dapper-looking older gentleman, across the room talking to her best friend, Celeste. Jack spotted her and winked. He turned back to Celeste who was standing next to him.

"Oh, there's Susan. Dave is here somewhere." Jack scanned the room for his old friend. "There he is. My God, Dave and Susan haven't changed a bit. Dave is a little grayer around the temples, but he still looks like a kid. You know, Dave will always be a special part of my life. I'll never forget the long nights that he and I spent in the bar and grill I used to run in Chicago. He was an earnest young man, full of idealism and determination. I would close the bar around 1:00 a.m. and Dave and I would stay up talking until 3:00, sometimes even 4:00. Those were hard times for those kids."

Celeste nodded in agreement. She was also impressed with how well Dave and Susan had done. "You were close to Dave. I think you were the one person he could really confide in."

Jack smiled. "I really didn't say much. I really didn't know what to say. Just listened mostly. I think that's what he needed people to do, just listen. Dave felt comfortable with me. I guess he saw me as a father figure. It was probably difficult to talk to men his own age. Remember, Dave was working with the labor unions. I imagine he didn't feel comfortable talking to most of the men there. I remember watching him move from hopeful excitement to denial and depression and then finally into resignation and acceptance."

"You two became pretty close. You spent a lot of time together, didn't you?" Celeste asked.

"Yeah, it became a kind of ritual. At least once a week, for about 3 years, Dave and I would burn the midnight oil."

"I remember," Celeste said.

Jack looked over at Susan. She was inspecting some of the gifts that had been laid out on the dining-room table. It's funny, but in all these years, he had never heard Susan and Dave quarrel. Susan always seemed so cool, so in control of every situation.

"Celeste, you were Susan's best friend. Did she mind all the late nights?" Jack asked.

"I don't think that Susan ever complained," Celeste answered.

Jack smiled. "Well, maybe she was glad he had someone to talk to. I do remember that he talked a lot about his parents. He wanted to be able to give them grandchildren." Jack recalled one of their early conversations when Dave was feeling especially low. He remembered the responsibility that Dave had felt to provide his parents with grandchildren, especially because they were getting older. Dave had once told him, "My folks are anxious to have grandchildren. You know, I really never thought about it before Susan and I began trying to have a family, but you want to be able to pass on your parents' genes. Now that I can't, I realize how important that is to me. When you have your choices taken away it becomes almost urgent."

"Jack, I guess you remember when they first began to consider the possibility of adoption," Celeste said.

"I remember it just like it was yesterday." Jack shook his head. "It's hard to believe that 10 years have passed so quickly."

Jack and Celeste made their way to the punch line. There was a large cardboard cutout caricature of a stork on the table. Celeste thought to herself that they hadn't changed the design on shower party favors for at least 20 years.

Jack served them both punch and continued, "It was a difficult decision for Dave. You know, they had already been under a doctor's care for 2 or 3 years. It was becoming clearer and clearer that their problem may be permanent. Dave was scared. His brother had adopted a child and that had helped to ease some of his fears. I think it was a weekday, in the summer about 8 or 9 years ago, when Dave called to tell me that they had adopted Cameron. I didn't see Dave too much after that. They moved to California a few months later. You know it's funny, but the girls really do resemble him and Susan."

Celeste nodded and looked at Jack. He had been a good friend to Dave. She wondered if she had been as good a friend to Susan.

Celeste glanced at Susan, now standing in the living room, and confessed to Jack, "It's strange that Susan and I never talk about those 3 years when they were trying to conceive. Maybe I'm afraid that Susan will tell me that I failed her as a best friend."

Jack shook his head and smiled. "You can't really believe that, Celeste. I'm sure you were very supportive."

Jack gave Celeste a warm hug cut short by a tap on his shoulder from Bill, who had just arrived. Bill and Jack moved effortlessly into joking conversation, and Celeste was thankful for a moment to herself. He didn't know the whole story. Celeste had gotten pregnant during the time that Susan and Dave were trying to conceive. She had decided to have an abortion. Although the memory made Celeste a little uncomfortable, she continued to recall how her relationship with Susan had changed.

Susan never said anything to me, but I knew that my abortion upset her. What was I supposed to do? I wasn't ready. She stopped talking to me about her infertility problems soon after that. Things got a little tense between Dave and Susan. I could feel it even when we talked on the phone. It was just an uncomfortable time. I often didn't know what to say.

Celeste silently remembered that some of their friends had already started to have children. She remembered the endless stream of shower invitations and wondered how Susan stood it. She also recalled how difficult it was for Susan to watch abusive parents deal with their children. Once when they were in a grocery store, she and Susan had seen a mother yell at her children. Susan had run out of the store, red-faced. Later she had told her that she did not know what emotion was stronger, the anger she felt toward the woman or the envy.

Celeste reminded herself that not every experience had been as heavy. It wasn't as though they never had light moments. There were times when Dave and Susan could actually joke around. She recalled how brave they both were to be able to laugh at the situation.

A lot of couples can't even talk about it, let alone laugh about it. Maybe that's what kept them sane through all of this. Celeste stifled a giggle when she remembered that they used to call Dave the "Dud Stud." It wasn't like they were hard to be around. They did their best to stay positive.

Celeste looked at some of the guests seated on a sofa that wrapped around a large television screen. The set was off, but the image triggered a memory of a similar scene 12 years ago. She remembered one night Dave, Susan, and her boyfriend were over at her place watching *Saturday Night Live*. The conversation had been somewhat guarded and everyone had been a little uptight.

Again, Celeste tamed an urge to laugh out loud as the memory became clearer. She remembered the skit with Dan Aykroyd and Gilda Radner as the Whiners. Ron Howard played the part of an infertility specialist and the Whiners were going to him for help because they couldn't get pregnant. It was a wonderful scene about how he was advising them to try artificial insemination and the two of them together whined, "Art-ifi-cial-insem-ina-tion?" The doctor said something like, "Well if you're not comfortable with that perhaps you should consider adoption." And the two Whiners looked at each other and exclaimed "Ad-op-ti-on—then it wouldn't be a Wh-in-er." Everyone had gotten hysterical. Celeste remembered that she had thought Dave and Susan were going to lose it. I guess it was sort of a release for them and for all of us really. Celeste suddenly felt sad. She missed those times.

She remembered the day Dave got the call that Cameron was going to be theirs. She even knew about Cameron before Susan did. She had arranged a baby shower for them that night. All of their friends were there. It was a magical night. There wasn't a dry eye in the place.

Celeste hoped that it made up for some of the agony that Susan had endured at other baby showers. She watched Susan as she chatted with four women who had formed a circle in the living room. Jack was right, Susan did look great. Celeste remembered that Susan was positively radiant the night of the shower. She had that glow that some women get when they are expecting. It was kind of like a pregnancy in fast forward. In one weekend they must have felt what all other couples have 9 months to think about.

A few weeks later Celeste had arranged another shower, much more organized. Everyone had given them a quilt that they had all been working on for months. No one had expected them to get a baby so soon. They only waited a little over a year for Cameron. Ava came a couple of years later. They really are a wonderful family. I guess its always darkest before the dawn, Celeste mused.

She and Susan did not spend as much time together as they both would like now that they were mothers. Celeste made a promise to herself that she would call Susan early next week to set up a lunch date. "No, I'll do it now," she said out loud. She followed Susan's voice to the dining room.

Celeste wondered if the shower was bringing up any old stuff for Susan too. When she found Susan standing alone, and saw the plaintive look on her face, she knew that it had.

"How are you doing?" Celeste asked softly.

"I'm really not sure. I guess I just needed some time out."

Celeste nodded and quietly left Susan alone with her thoughts.

THE DECISION TO CONCEIVE

Susan and Dave had known most of the people there since the time when the thought of having children was just a pleasant abstraction. Susan remembered that in the first 8 years of their marriage, they had not wanted any encumbrances. They hadn't wanted to be tied down in any way. A really serious discussion of having children didn't come until they were just about ready to try. She thought back to the early years of their marriage. It seemed that there were several times that one of them was more ready than the other, and they discussed it briefly from time to time. It was a kind of back and forth. Neither of them ever said, "Forget it—no way am I ever considering this." They had just accepted that the other was not ready and waited. They had both been busy with their careers and had traveled extensively. Throughout the 1970s, they had been involved in a variety of political organizations and political work. The older they got the more they realized just how big a responsibility it really was and it became easier to defer.

Susan looked over at Connie and Sheldon, a young newlywed couple. Susan had heard that they both had decided not to have children. It was a lifestyle choice that Susan respected but could not relate to. They look a little lost, too, Susan thought. These functions must be difficult for couples without children—even if the choice is theirs.

She remembered the evening that she and Dave first admitted that they both had been experiencing a faint and indistinct feeling of dissatisfaction with their lives. Dave initiated the conversation.

"Susan, you know we're almost 30 years old. We're both working and making a little money. We've done a lot of traveling, been and lived in a lot of places, even different countries. We've pursued many activities. I mean, we have done a lot of things, you know, I think we've lived pretty full lives. It may sound strange"—he paused briefly and continued—"I don't know how it sounds, but I think our lives are beginning to feel a little empty. Maybe this is just a convoluted way of saying that our time may be running out. Maybe we should have kids. I can't imagine the idea of not having kids and continuing to live the lives we have been leading. It might be more rewarding to share what we have now with children. I want to be young enough to actually enjoy activities with our kids." Susan agreed. Only a few months later, they began their struggle to conceive.

Susan overheard some men on the patio joking about the unreliable nature of condoms. She smiled to herself when she thought of what she called the "incredible irony of their situation," and how much it is likely to be similar to the others.

For 10 years they had been extremely conscientious. They were so careful about birth control and they probably did not need to be. She recalled that in their lighter moments she and Dave would joke about how much money they had spent over the years on contraceptives. She also remembered being tormented by self-recriminations, wondering if they had made a mistake by waiting so long to start a family. She could almost hear the familiar litany that always began with, "Maybe, if we had started a little earlier we may have been able to give birth to our own child." Susan took comfort in the knowledge that they had done the right thing by waiting. Anyway, they both were probably infertile at 23.

The Doctor

Susan's thoughts were interrupted again. This time a familiar-sounding voice caused her to turn and face the entryway. She saw Dr. Martin Anderson's profile in the doorway and she suddenly understood why her mother had warned her about seeing an infertility specialist who was a mutual friend.

"High fences make good neighbors," her mother had said. "Do you want everybody to know your business?"

Susan had laughed at her mother's reaction back then. But she had to admit, it did feel a little uncomfortable to see Martin socially. She hadn't seen him for a couple of years. It was a chance meeting in a department store. She had been glad to see him then. But in this particular context, the best she could manage was a smile and a small gesture with her hand that could only be described as a half-hearted attempt at a wave.

Dr. Anderson's wife, Janet, recognized Susan immediately.

"Martin, weren't Susan and Dave Jones patients of yours?" Janet asked.

"Yes, Susan and Dave are a great couple. I treated them both for 3 years and I got to know them pretty well. They were great to work with because they had great attitudes." Dr. Anderson returned Susan's less than enthusiastic wave. He wondered if she would approach him. Probably not, he thought to himself. I guess this situation could be a little uncomfortable for her.

Janet saw Susan disappear quickly to the other room. Susan's reaction made her a bit uncomfortable. Although Janet thought that Susan should show a little more appreciation for all Martin's efforts, she did not say anything to her husband.

"What was the problem, Martin?"

"They were what we call subfertile. That is, maybe with another partner they may have been able to conceive. The way the wall of Susan's uterus was lined made her unable to hold a child. Also the term subfertile was so much easier to digest. It sounded less conclusive, less brutal than infertile. At that point in time, I thought that there was a small chance that they could conceive. In retrospect, maybe I did them a disservice, but it didn't seem wise to demoralize them at a time when their mental state was such a crucial component of their treatment."

Susan had reentered the room, but did not look over at Janet or her husband. Janet tried to temper her feelings of animosity.

"Martin, I'm sure you did what you thought was best," Janet said, a little more emphatically than she meant to.

Dr. Anderson gave his wife an affectionate look and continued, "Dave had an extremely low sperm count and low motility. I checked them both out immediately. Some of my colleagues hesitate to treat the man early in treatment and I strongly disagree with that practice. It's just not fair to the woman. Of course, that was 15 years ago. Things have really changed. They came in every 3 months or so. At first, I prescribed all the typical treatments for Dave: cool baths and loose underwear. I remembered he laughed at the suggestion of the underwear. But the next time he came in, I noticed he had made the change to boxer short."

"Did either one of them have surgery?" Janet asked.

"Dave insisted on the varicoelectomy. At that time it was a painful procedure designed to cool down the sperm in order to increase its production. It knocked him out for quite a while, 2 or 3 weeks."

After 25 years of marriage, Janet had never lost interest in her husband's work. She asked, "What kind of treatment did you use on Susan?"

"The lining of Susan's cervix did not have proper consistency. It was difficult for a fertilized egg to attach. I started her on a fertility drug called Chlomid. She was on it steadily for 2 years. It was really a long shot. It was simply a way of enhancing the lining in the off chance that Dave could produce viable sperm. After 3 years of treatment, I suggested what was for them at that time a last-ditch effort, artificial insemination. They considered it and then decided against it. I know it was a difficult call for them both. There were some new treatments some of my colleagues were experimenting with, but Susan and Dave were exhausted. I felt that Susan was becoming dissatisfied with my care. She probably thought I was not being as aggressive as I could have been. It happens a lot. The couples are so desperate for a child, they look for anything or anyone to blame."

"I guess you must be used to that by now," Janet said.

"It's never really easy. But you do get used to it. Over the last year of their treatment, I tried to let them down as gently as possible. I saw little hope for them. I mentioned adoption in passing a number of times. Near the end, I think that Susan knew what I was trying to do."

Janet suddenly felt guilty for her early feelings of animosity. She had been watching Susan interact with her daughter, now seated on Susan's lap. They look so natural together.

"How old were they? Susan and Dave look so young."

"They were both in their early 30s when they first came in. At that time, there was this sort of panic about the 'biological clock' and time running out. Of course, today, so much has changed from a technological standpoint. Women in their 60s have delivered healthy children. But back then, there was a strong sense of urgency for many of the couples I treated."

"At least this case had a happy ending," Janet replied.

"One way or another, couples seem to find a way to cope, eventually." Dr. Anderson was happy that Susan and Dave had found their answer.

Dave's Story

Seeing Dr. Anderson and the others under one roof was just as unsettling for Dave as it was for Susan. The vividness of some of the memories jolted him as well. Dave looked across the room, past the stack of torn wrapping paper, at Susan. He could tell that she was remembering, too. He tried to imagine how she would feel if she knew that he still wondered what a child conceived from his own body would look like. He closed his eyes and tried to shut out the thought. But he couldn't. He did not like having these feelings. He knew that these feelings did not seriously affect his relationship with his two adopted children. But as satisfied as he was with the decisions that Susan and he had made, he was still aware that they were not his own flesh and blood.

It's just a tiny part of him that was aware that they were not his own. He couldn't help wondering what his own children would have looked like. As much as he tried to fight the emotion, if he was honest, he would have to admit that he was still envious of people who really do see their own physical features in their children. Maybe it's biological, this urge to pass on your own genes to leave something of yourself behind.

The decision to adopt did not come as easily for Dave as it did for Susan. He still had a vivid memory of a young boy named Andy whom he encountered while working with emotionally disturbed kids in his native Scotland. Andy was a particularly difficult child. Dave remembered isolating the boy and talking to him. The child was very upset. Dave had tried to reassure him. "You're a good kid. We value you and we like you, even if we sometimes do not like your behavior." Dave will never forget the boy's tragic response.

"I am not good, I am bad." Dave asked him what he meant.

"It's obvious, isn't it? I'm adopted. My parents did not want me."

The incident left a permanent mark on Dave. It raised doubts about his own ability to be able to care for an adopted child properly. Would what he had to offer be enough? The question continued to haunt him. Maybe that's why he reacted the way he did to the call from the agency.

Dave heard Susan's laugh from the across the room and began to feel a familiar pang of shame as he recalled the event. He had been working out of town a lot, but this particular day he had happened to be home. It was around midmorning when the telephone began to ring. Dave remembered he had slept in late. The telephone may have rung earlier that morning. He wasn't really sure. He had been half in and half out of sleep. This time there was no way of ignoring it. It continued to ring loudly as Dave made his way down the stairs to the telephone. The voice on the other end sounded unfamiliar.

"Who is this?" Dave had asked immediately.

"Mr. Jones, this is Ms. Lopez, the social worker assigned to your case. We may have a baby girl for you."

There was a sense of urgency in her voice. She knew that Susan and Dave were planning to leave for Europe the next day.

Dave calmly asked, "Well, we have these tickets to Paris and we are leaving tomorrow. Can't we see her when we get back?"

He remembered the long pause and the tone of voice that indicated that Ms. Lopez was a little taken aback at his response.

"No, Mr. Jones, we have to place this baby immediately. You know the decision has not been made yet. It has not been finalized. You are one of two couples that we are considering, and I just want to tell you that you might get a phone call tomorrow, which is the day I know you are planning to leave."

Of course, he called Susan immediately. They did not travel at all that year or even the next 3. He was still not sure if Susan had ever completely forgiven him for trying to postpone Cameron's arrival.

She had said to him at the time, "My God, Dave, how could you hesitate for even 1 second? This is the moment of our lives!"

They had not spoken of it since.

Dave had a horrible vision of Cameron being given to someone else. He shuddered at the thought of their lives without her.

Susan's Story

Some of the guests were starting to leave. Susan suddenly felt drained. She hadn't thought of the time before the girls in such a long time, she realized. Maybe it's a good thing to remember.

Mary interrupted Susan, offering her a glass of punch.

"Susan, are you okay?"

Susan laughed. "Yeah, I'm fine. You know it's been a long time since I've been to one of these things."

Mary seemed relieved. "Susan, were you the one with the problem or was it Dave?"

"We were both what they called subfertile, back then. We may have been able to conceive with other partners, but the combination of both our conditions made it next to impossible for us to conceive together." Susan could tell from the look on Mary's face that her situation was not the same.

"And what about you two, Mary?"

Mary's voice was barely audible. "It's me."

This time Susan did not hesitate to put her arm around Mary. She still could not find words to comfort the woman. Suddenly she felt sympathy for many of her own friends who must have faced a similar dilemma 12 years before.

Susan couldn't help but wonder what would have happened if her situation had been different. What if it had only been Dave or worse what if it had only been her with the problem? Would they have been able to hold it together? In a way it was sort of made easy, because they both had things wrong with them. She could imagine how natural, how easy, it would be to feel anger toward the infertile partner.

Toward the end it had been difficult enough. Three years of monthly highs and lows. Susan remembered how the emotional cycles fit in with the menstrual cycles when they were trying to conceive. Every month she read all sorts of things into minor messages from her body that would convince her every month that "this was it." "My breasts are just a little bit sorer this month!" or "This cramping doesn't feel quite the way it normally does." God, every month I put myself through such torture, thinking that this time I really was pregnant, and then, of course, my period would come.

It didn't help that Susan had such irregular menstrual cycles. She had become obsessed with the calendar. Every month the countdown would begin again. "Only 22 days until my period might or might not start. Oh, now it's only 21." She had lived for the calendar. No sooner had one period ended then she would literally start counting the days until the next one. She would always become so depressed after the bleeding started. It was painful to remember. Especially the time that she was so very, very sure. Her period was even later than usual. She had bought a home pregnancy kit, and it came out positive. She was so excited that she trembled as she dialed the doctor's number to make an appointment. She remembered the elation she felt, thinking, this is really it! Even the pregnancy kit tells me I am.

She could not remember much after the leaving the doctor's office, except the words, "You're not pregnant," that kept turning over and over in her mind. It had been a very low time her life.

She could not help thinking that if the situation had been different, maybe she and Dave might not have made it. She refused to consider the possibility. But she could not suppress a strong feeling of relief.

They had their own problems. Susan drifted back to the many times she accused Dave of not caring.

I was doing so much grieving. I was so obsessed and in my mind I thought he wasn't sharing an equal share of my burden. I wanted him to hurt like I did. I wanted to pull him down with me. I felt so hopeless. I was just so consumed by my grief. I guess I needed a lot of sympathy.

Dave's response was always the same. "Susan, you don't give me any room to do my own grieving. You're doing it all for me."

Susan had never asked Dave if he had resented her obsession. She knew it was hard for him too. Men just don't talk comfortably about the things that really matter. But even now she wondered if it was just a cop-out. Dave had tried to cope in his own way. In all fairness, Dave had felt that she was just so low. She thought he felt he needed to do whatever he could to try and bring her out of this and that probably included little hopeful things like, "Well, you know, maybe next time."

Susan looked lovingly across the room at her husband as he helped their daughter, Cameron, with her sweater. Susan thought that maybe it was because of the hard times that their marriage had grown stronger. It's something they rose above. In many ways, they were pulled together over it. She knew that she had become more sensitive to his needs after that.

THE FUTURE

Susan and Mary were standing alone now. Susan wanted to leave Mary with some words of comfort, but she knew the inconsolable nature of Mary's grief. She wanted to tell Mary that she must do whatever she needed to do go get through this. She wanted to tell her how almost 5 years of obsession, pain, and depression had been released immediately when Susan had arrived at her own solution, adoption. Susan had never had any feelings of remorse once she and Dave had made their choice. She could not imagine that Dave felt any differently. They both had come to terms with the fact that this was how they were going to have their family. Once they held Cameron for the first time, and a few years later Ava, it was like none of the pain had really happened, well . . . almost.

Although many people, her friends and family, her doctor, and even her church, may tell her that they have the answer and that they know what is best for her, the solution is for Mary and her husband to find. Whatever path they take, it must be their own.

Susan wanted to tell Mary all of this as soon as possible.

"Mary, are you free for lunch next week?"

"I'd love it. How about Wednesday afternoon?" Mary seemed relieved by the invitation.

"Sounds great. I'll call you tomorrow."

RELEVANT CONCEPTS

biological urge/biological clock
childlessness
infertility
social support
solutions/choices
unmet expectations

DISCUSSION QUESTIONS

1. There are topics that Susan, Dave, and Celeste never discuss. What are they? Is it important to discuss these issues? Why or why not?

2. Susan and Dave were trying to conceive at a time when our society pressured women to have children by the age of 30. Today, what obvious and subtle messages do men and women receive about having children or about childlessness? Where do these messages come from (e.g., religion, families, medical establishment), and how do they act to disenfranchise or enfranchise couples experiencing infertility?

3. What disenfranchising messages did Susan and Dave receive from others or situations?

4. In what ways did Susan and Dave disenfranchise themselves from others while experiencing infertility?

5. How have technological advances for infertility acted to disenfranchise or enfranchise couples experiencing infertility?

SUGGESTED READINGS

Franklin, R. R., & Rockman, D. K. (1990). *In pursuit of fertility.* New York: Holt.

Glazer, E. S. (1990). *The long awaited stork: A guide to parenting after infertility.* New York: Lexington.

Goldfarb, H. A. (1995). *Overcoming infertility.* New York: Wiley.

Hanson, M. F. (1994). *Infertility: The emotional journey.* Minneapolis: Deaconess Press.

Luebberman, M. (1995). *Coping with miscarriage: A simple guide to emotional and physical health.* Rocklin, CA: Prima.

Lauersen, N. H., & Bouchez, C. (1991). *Getting pregnant: What couples need to know right now.* New York: Ballantine.

Silber, S. J. (1991). *How to get pregnant with the new technology.* New York: Warner Books.

Treiser, S., & Levinson, R. K. (1994). *A woman doctor's guide to infertility.* New York: Hyperion.

6 *Coping With Adolescent Cancer: One Family's Experience*

Deborah S. Ballard-Reisch
University of Nevada, Reno

Jennifer Price
Lakeland, Florida

In May of 1986, my sister Jennifer (the second author of this chapter) was diagnosed with acute lymphoblastic leukemia. This type of leukemia accounts for 90% of all childhood leukemia, with the best prognosis for children between 2 and 14 years of age (American Cancer Society, 1991). Jennifer was 15 years old. The diagnosis of her leukemia initiated a family crisis that is only now, 10 years later, approaching resolution. In June 1994, Jennifer was considered cured. This is her story and the stories of our parents, with myself (the first author and Jennifer's oldest sister) acting as historian and narrator of their stories.[1] From our discussions, three common issues arose during my family's experiences with Jennifer's leukemia and provide the focus of this chapter: (a) communication within the health care context, specifically information gathering, input into decision making, and communication with hospital personnel, (b) reactions to social support efforts, and (c) communication within the family.

COMMUNICATION WITHIN THE HEALTH CARE CONTEXT

Within the health care setting, acquiring information about the illness, participation in decision making, and communication with health care

[1]My story is not included here because I experienced most of this crisis from my home 3,000 miles away.

providers are extremely important as the patient and family cope with the crisis of a life-threatening illness.

Information Gathering

The extent to which patients and family members engage in information gathering varies widely, ranging from ignorance to vigilance to suppressing undesirable information. These approaches may also change throughout the course of treatment and were evident in Jennifer's case.

My sister and our parents differed greatly in their desire for information throughout Jennifer's treatment for cancer. When asked how much information she wanted about leukemia when she was first diagnosed, Jennifer replied, "None. I didn't want to believe I had it." Our parents, however, demonstrated a vigilant approach to coping with the stress. When asked how much information they wanted, Mom replied, "Everything you could find out about it." Dad replied, "More than I previously would have ever dreamed I would want to know."

Their patterns changed as treatment progressed. Once the initial shock wore off and the treatment program was underway, Jennifer's pattern changed to one of vigilance. She reflected, "Later I wanted to know and I wanted everyone else to know." Dad's pattern also changed. He stated, "As I went along, there was more and more things that came up that was scary, that I began to wonder if I really did want to know all about leukemia . . . I really blocked out the bad things. I didn't want to know about side-effects. You worry enough, it's a constant 24-hour worry. I didn't want to know her kidneys was goin' bad or her liver. I wanted to hear all the good things—positives about leukemia." Mom maintained her vigilant approach to information. She commented, "You want to know everything there is to know and where you stand and so on. Never back down from it . . . and I still never got all the information that I really wanted."

Participation in Decision Making

In the context of leukemia management, the family and patient often have little choice and very little input into treatment decisions,[2] especially if they agree to participate in a clinical treatment trial. After diagnosis and while exploring treatment alternatives, neither my sister nor our parents felt that

[2]The unique characteristics of the state of the leukemia treatment in the 1980s and 1990s make it impossible to integrate the leukemia experience into a participative decision-making framework. Within the medical establishment, there are few alternatives available for leukemia patients.

they had much chance to be involved in decision making. They were unaware of options; the hospital didn't offer any and the urgency of the situation led them to believe they had no choices and no time to look for alternatives.

Only Mom indicated that she didn't feel prepared to be involved in decision making at first, but she then responded strongly to her perception of her lack of choice: "In the very beginning . . . I was totally numb and we were informed that you do not have a decision. You had to sign papers that they would choose the manner of treatment and so on. You just didn't really have a choice." Dad remembered more of a collaborative approach within the context of limited choices:

> They kinda had a protocol they went by and for her type, I think we had two choices: doing it [chemotherapy] all at one time, or spreading it out over a lengthy time. We asked Jennifer, if I remember right, and went with the "let's get it over with" protocol. Once we made that decision, it was pretty much out of our hands.

Jennifer felt that she had no choice:

> I wasn't allowed to decide whether I wanted this or not . . . They [medical personnel and parents] told me what was gonna happen: when, where, why, and how . . . There wasn't any [decision] to make. Your protocol was how it was and you couldn't refuse treatment.

Although they did not feel involved in the decision-making process, both parents felt that Jennifer received the best treatment possible. Mom summarized, "I do believe she had the best program she could have had." Dad felt that involvement in decision making was "adequate, appropriate."

Communication With Medical Personnel

Our parents were less satisfied with actual interaction with medical personnel. With respect to interaction with doctors, Dad found them "tight-lipped—you had to really pry out of them to get what you wanted to know . . . I think they evaded or used terms that you're not really sure of." Mom had a similar perspective:

> They [doctors] don't want to talk to you, they don't want to take the time, to answer all your questions and so on. They are fine right at the beginning but then it's more or less, oh, you should know this or you should know that type of thing . . . as things came up, they would come in and give us a short briefing but you never got really any chance to ask too many questions. You never got the time with the doctors; you'd get a quick something and half the things you would ask, they're out the door before you could get answers.

She concluded, "You could ask anything you wanted to if you could run somebody down." This lack of time to ask doctors questions was also reflected in Dad's perspective. He said, "At times, you might have had to go back and ask two or three times. I think they were pretty busy at certain times with other patients and they really didn't have time to give you the full attention you really wanted." Jennifer agreed that "information wasn't volunteered, you had to ask . . . they [medical personnel] didn't want you to get down about it." Her story reflects the important role Mom played in asking questions for her, which allowed Jennifer to be a passive recipient of information. She didn't have to ask questions because she knew Mom would. It comforted her to know that Mom "knew everything," that "Mom asked everything I wanted to know."

Even though the process of gathering information was at times frustrating, Jennifer and our parents had a great deal of confidence in the medical staff, and staff reactions had a significant impact on family reactions. Dad stated, "He [doctor] seemed so confident it made me feel confident so I think that's why I really didn't ask too many questions. 'She's doin' fine, we're happy' and that made me happy." Jennifer also felt that her doctor cared about her and had her best interests at heart.

SOCIAL SUPPORT

In addition to information gathering, decision making, and communication with health care professionals, social support plays an important role in the ability of patients and their families to cope with cancer. Social support is not only important to the patient, it is fundamental in assisting the family in coping with the crisis (see, e.g., Figley & McCubbin, 1983; Rait & Lederberg, 1989). Support from spouse, family, friends, and the primary care physician significantly impacts a parent's ability to adjust to a child's cancer (Morrow, Hoagland, & Carnrike, 1981).

Its importance to patient outcomes has led many hospitals to attempt to formalize support networks for patients and their families. Unfortunately, the imposition of social support on families does not always have the desired effect.

Other Cancer Patients and Their Families

It was common for the hospital staff, particularly nurses and the social worker, to encourage parents of children with cancer to seek out other parents whose children had just been diagnosed, and to encourage cancer patients to interact with newly diagnosed cancer patients. My family expressed strong reactions to this support. Dad stated:

> When we first got there, there were a couple of parents that came and tried to talk with us. You've got your mind everywhere but right there on that conversation and really, you're just worried, right at that time, about Jennifer and, ah, you don't want, and that might be hard to say, but you're not really worried about anyone else right at that particular time.

He felt that their privacy had been "invaded" at a time when they needed to deal with the emotional shock of the diagnosis. He concluded, "You want to be left alone initially to just go through it by yourself because the initial shock is not over."

Mom concurred. She felt that the least helpful method of support came from "people [parents of children with cancer], they [social worker/coordinator of the support group] pushed on me down there at the beginning. I think that's the worst thing in the world to do to someone. They need their time and space at first."

Jennifer also responded strongly to this type of imposed support:

> I hated it. I know that's bad, but if I wanna go and talk to people about the illness, then that should be my prerogative. I don't like going to people I don't know when they first get diagnosed 'cause I don't think anybody wants to have people they don't know when you're first diagnosed. I think it's wrong to be pushed into that. If I know 'em, it'd be different and if I didn't like bein' bombarded when I was first diagnosed and, and you just don't. I don't think you should do that. They think it's supportive but . . .

Clearly, for our family the imposition of social support from strangers, even those who had recently gone through something similar, was uncomfortable. All three spoke of the need for time and space to come to terms with their feelings prior to intervention from others. Interestingly, all found such support helpful later. Jennifer recounted a story of the importance of having a friend her age going through the same thing she was:

> It really helped to be around people the same way as you are, because they're coping with the same thing, and if you were in school, people don't understand; people make fun of you, but if you're there, in the hospital, with, like friends your age and stuff, it's easier to cope.

A real camaraderie developed between the children with cancer. Jennifer recalled the importance of this connection, particularly at tough times. The most difficult experience for her was losing her hair, a common side-effect of chemotherapy. One special friend who had gone through chemotherapy prior to Jennifer made that bearable for her, using humor to combat their fear. Jennifer reflected:

> Just bein' with Sandy, we used to joke about it 'cause she was already through almost everything. She was getting her hair back as I was losin' mine . . . I remember pullin' my hair out, clumps and clumps boy! She would just grab on. At that time [in the hospital], we laughed. If it had happened anywhere else, probably not.

Jennifer summarized the importance of being around people who were going through similar experiences and the anger she sometimes felt toward those who claimed to understand what she was going through. She said, "We knew what each other were going through and others said they did, that they know how we felt, but they didn't." Words of understanding from a fellow cancer patient may be reassuring. These same words, however, from a friend or staff member can elicit anger and disgust (Rowland, 1989).

Our parents found interaction with other parents helpful. Dad saw them as a major source of supplemental information about how to cope and what to expect with Jennifer. However, he still had reservations: "I didn't want to rely too much on that either because they [other parents] could just bring in some things that would just have you lookin' to see if you could see that in Jennifer."

Mom's feelings were similar: "You got more information from other people that had been through things than you did from your doctors and your nurses. People tried to work together that way." She felt that many parents got to know one another because of their similar experiences and developed a sort of informal support network where they would ask and answer questions and "help you out with your feelings because they had already been there."

Doctors

There was a notable lack of communication about feelings and coping with the doctors. Although both parents indicated that the doctors were the people they approached first and most often when they wanted information, they did not share feelings with them. About her primary physician, Jennifer concluded, "He'd be blunt and to the point, like wham-bam see you later. He's not personable but I knew he had other people to contend with."

Nurses

Nurses were important sources of social support for all parties. On one occasion, Mom was very concerned about how Jennifer was responding to treatment. She recalled that she had "badgered the doctors into performing a bone marrow." The nurses on shift were so worried, they stayed after hours to find out the results of the tests. When they came back okay, one of the nurses hugged Mom. That the nurses cared and that they stayed meant a great deal to her.

Dad also had high regard for the nurses: "Our nurses couldn't have been any better; we could talk to them on a daily basis. I felt that was a part of the recovery process, too, for Jennifer and myself."

Jennifer felt that her nurses were understanding and caring. She could talk to them "just about it bein' a bummer and just anything."

Friends

All three found friends to be important sources of social support and coping assistance. Emotional and instrumental support (House, 1981) were the most important types of assistance for both parents. Mom talked primarily to two women friends for emotional support, one of them, a coworker.

Dad found support outside the family to be the most helpful. The majority of his support came from clients and coworkers. A valuable message Dad got from his bosses was that he didn't have to worry about his job. He said, "That was one of the biggest morale boosters, that I could concentrate on Jennifer and I didn't have to worry about losin' my job."

The need to provide financial support often collides with the need to provide emotional support. An individual cannot be both at work, earning a living for the family, and at the hospital caring for a child. Although he did not have to totally sacrifice one for the other, Dad felt a great deal of empathy for those who did not have the job flexibility he had: "I was glad I was there for her, that I had that opportunity, because I did see some of the parents didn't have that opportunity and I feel sorry for them." Mom added, "If they have unsupportive employers, families are doomed."

Friends from her life before leukemia were also important to Jennifer. She felt that her friends had trouble dealing with the reality of her illness, as well as having a lot of questions, so she tried to keep her communication with them spontaneous and open. About her friends, Jennifer said:

> Sometimes they would just ask—some people were shy so I made it clear I didn't care . . . Some of 'em were scared and didn't want to be around 'cause they didn't know what they were getting themselves into. I think they were scared of losing me.

Jennifer didn't have to try to maintain contact with her friends. She said, "They sought me out . . . they were always there."

One of the most frustrating experiences for my family involved dealing with people who did not understand or accept the nature or severity of Jennifer's illness. Two examples from Mom's story illustrate this point.

First, during her chemotherapy treatment, Jennifer fluctuated between vigor and weakness. Frustrated with her inconsistent behavior, one of her teachers accused her of "faking her illness." Second, shortly after the illness was diagnosed, one of her good friends told her that her mother had decided she could no longer be around Jennifer as she might "catch leukemia from her." The inflexibility and lack of knowledge on the part of both Jennifer's teacher and her friend's mother infuriated Mom. She concluded, "People just don't know how to deal with ill children and their families. There ought to be a class to teach them!"

Summary

Our family found support conducive to coping in many traditional places, such as support groups, nurses, and friends. However, doctors, although involved in treatment tasks (instrumental support), were not a direct source of emotional or informational support. Also, the hospital's attempts to force social support in the form of other parents of children with cancer, and the children themselves, before my family was ready, were not appreciated. Mom, Dad, and Jennifer clearly underscored the need for a "coming to terms" period, when they could deal with the shock of the cancer diagnosis prior to intervention from supportive strangers. In addition to support from those outside the family, communication, coping, and support within the family are important to illness management.

FAMILY STRENGTHS AND STRESS

Family members struggling with a crisis event may emerge less healthy and more vulnerable than before, or they may move toward increased health, maturity, and growth (McCubbin, Cauble, & Patterson, 1982). Individual coping patterns and communication within the family are strong determinants of the family's ability to manage the crisis.

Individual Coping Strategies

Our parents felt that the family really pulled together during Jennifer's illness, and coping strategies really helped meet one another's needs. Mom described her feelings: "You start out with numbness, thinking the worst, and then as things progress, you begin to cope because there's nothing else you can do but cope and you try to make things go as well as they can go." Just as in information gathering, Mom coped by being vigilant:

> I was just there and, ah, probably overprotecting a lot of times because if I was there nothing was gonna happen. Things were gonna be okay and that went to the extent of checking her umpteen times a night. Jennifer said I

lived with my hand on her face. I was totally involved; she was not left alone for any reason. I held the bedpan for the 36 hours she threw up and the whole bit and if she needed something, I made sure she got it . . . I didn't want anybody doing anything with her that I didn't know exactly what was going on. There was nothing done that I wasn't involved with.

This vigilance had both an irritating and soothing effect on Jennifer. The complexity of her dependency on Mom is clear:

> Mom was the bad and good guy. She let me take out my frustrations. She was very irritable too. She irritated me too. She always had this positive attitude when sometimes I just didn't want to hear it . . . She was grumpy and she made me grumpy and would, like my lips would be chapped and I was wantin' her there and she'd be like, "Let me cream your heels," constantly. I wanted her there but not always doing something.

As Jennifer put it, Mom "was my punching bag but also a soft pillow."

As noted earlier, Dad coped primarily by relying on his friends outside the family. However, it was also important for him to "be there for Jennifer." However, he had particular problems with one side-effect of Jennifer's chemotherapy. Overall, he said, the side-effects "did not bother me, she took it so well, at first she cried [when she started to lose her hair] and you just wanted to cry with her, but it didn't bother me . . . But when she got sick I'd leave the room. I just couldn't handle seein' her sick." Here, nonverbal communication provided an important cue for Dad. Jennifer shook her foot a certain way a couple of minutes prior to vomiting, so whenever he saw her foot move in that way, Dad would leave the room.

Religion. For both parents, prayer and faith in God were, and continue to be, fundamental parts of their coping strategies. Dad viewed prayer as his strongest coping mechanism: "To this day, I pray for her every day; you've got to leave it in His hands." Mom saw things similarly: "Prayer was the biggest thing. The power of prayer, it makes a difference." Mom told of some initial difficulty going to church without Jennifer when the leukemia was first diagnosed. She felt that something was missing when Jennifer wasn't there. When Jennifer was well enough to go back to church on Sundays, Mom felt back in balance again. For Jennifer, however, prayer was not a part of her coping strategy.

Communication

There was little verbal communication in the family about the leukemia. Jennifer perceived communication as spontaneous. "If someone had something to say, they said it . . . we'd just all the sudden be sittin' at the dinner table and talk." She felt that her personal communication patterns had a lot to do with what she was going through at the time, and that overall, she became more blunt and direct in interactions with our parents. "They [parents] got more relaxed, the way I could talk to 'em, 'cause I was very, very, very moody and they knew it and I could just say really anything I wanted."

Because of her illness, Mom saw Jennifer as the person who set the rules regarding talk:

> Jennifer didn't like to talk about it a lot and I would listen when she would say things. I didn't try to hide anything and if I had something to say, I said it but, as far as really discussing it, she was never into a lot of discussion.

Dad felt his own reluctance to talk about the illness: "We would talk some but I really didn't want to talk about it." He explained this reluctance as well as his need to seek support from outside the family: "I just felt the people inside [the family] was feeling the same way I was and they didn't want anything negative and generally you can pick up positive things from outside your family." Mom validated this perspective: "Your family is too closely involved sometimes and somebody outside can be a little more objective than the ones going through it."

Although there wasn't a lot of verbal communication, Mom felt the family communicated their closeness by just being there for each other. Jennifer put her views of communication within the family into a life stage perspective: "Communication is better now. I'm not an ornery little child anymore. I grew up. There's a difference when you were younger and older anyway. You can't really compare that—from a teenager to a more mature adult."

Fluctuations between closeness and distance occurred during Jennifer's illness. Dad's view was that, "at first I think it strengthens you, pulls you together, and then things happen as you go and I think it pulls you apart." Mom also viewed change over the course of the illness. "At the time [of the diagnosis], I think it strengthened it [communication]. I don't think it's as strong as it was. Everyone pulled together; now I don't see all that, but then, yes." Dad attempted to explain some of the tension:

> There's times it's still there. When she gets a fever, or she goes to get her bone marrow or her spinal test, even today. And I would think probably until the end or whatever, it'll always be a big worry. You ask why she got it. They can't answer why she got it and in the back of my mind is if they say she's cured why can't she get it again like she did before and that still bothers me.

Overall, my sister and our parents feel that their experience has brought them closer. Mom noted, "My family was the biggest support." Dad commented, "We pulled through. I think we did a good job." Jennifer added, "Our relationships are stronger now. It pulled us together."

CONCLUSION

The stories told by Jennifer and our parents highlight the importance of quality communication and strong and diverse social support systems when coping with a crisis. Support within and outside the family was significant for each of them. For our parents, support from each other, family, friends, nurses, and the physician were especially important. For Jennifer, the support of family, friends who had gone through similar experiences, and her doctor and nurses were instrumental in her keeping a positive attitude throughout her treatment.

However, the need to communicate effectively and comprehensively is underscored by the frustration our parents felt when they tried to get information from doctors. Charges of evasiveness and a lack of time led to dissatisfaction with communication. In this case, the positive outcomes and the trust our parents felt in the doctor overcame their exasperation. However, the experience of having a child with a life-threatening illness is stressful enough without having to deal with an underresponsive medical establishment.

As for Jennifer, she is philosophical about her experience with leukemia:

> I'm glad I was able to have it, in a way, because I appreciate life more and you look at things in a different perspective than you did beforehand. You think nothing can happen to you. I still don't think anything happened to me if you want to know the honest truth. I just think it's a way of life.

RELEVANT CONCEPTS

adolescent cancer
coping strategies
illness management
personal control
social support
stigmatization

DISCUSSION QUESTIONS

1. How might Jennifer's age make a difference in the family's experience?
2. Discuss helpful and unhelpful types and sources of support received by family members and how these might change from diagnosis to treatment to recovery.
3. In what ways were Jennifer and her family stigmatized through the course of her illness? How were they empowered?

4. Jennifer's parents noted that they felt the doctors were evasive and would not take time to discuss their concerns with them. What are some reasons for the doctors' avoidance of communication? How might health care providers be affected by caring for adolescents with cancer? How might this impact their communication with the patient and the patient's family? What might be the impact of this evasiveness on the patient and family?

ACKNOWLEDGMENT

The authors would like to thank Linda Wagner for her research assistance throughout the preparation of this manuscript.

REFERENCES/SUGGESTED READINGS

American Cancer Society. (1991). *Cancer facts and figures.* Atlanta: Author.

Figley, C., & McCubbin, H. (1983). *Stress and the family: Coping with catastrophe* (Vol. 3). New York: Brunner/Mazel.

House, J. S. (1981). *Work stress and social support.* Reading, MA: Addison-Wesley.

McCubbin, H., Cauble, A., & Patterson, J. (1982). *Family stress, coping and social support.* Springfield, IL: Thomas.

Morrow, G., Hoagland, A., & Carnrike, C. (1981). Social support and parental adjustment to pediatric cancer. *Journal of Consulting and Clinical Psychology, 49,* 763–765.

Rait, D., & Lederberg, M. (1989). The family of the cancer patient. In J. C. Holland & J. H. Rowland (Eds.), *Handbook of psychooncology: Psychological care of the patient with cancer* (pp. 585–597). New York: Oxford University Press.

Rowland, J. H. (1989). Interpersonal resources: Coping. In J. C. Holland & J. H. Rowland (Eds.), *Handbook of psychooncology: Psychological care of the patient with cancer* (pp. 44–57). New York: Oxford University Press.

7 *Divorce Mediation: Balancing the Scales of Justice?*[1]

Jill E. Rudd
Cleveland State University

Daniel P. Joyce
Cleveland Mediation Center

Sarah and Ed have been married for 15 years. They have three boys, ages 14, 10, and 5. They own a home in Ohio valued at $140,000 (a mortgage balance of $20,000), a 17-foot boat, and an investment portfolio valued at nearly $20,000 that Ed has managed for the last 5 years. Ed is an independent consultant who works primarily with teacher unions in bargaining contracts. He has earned an average of $80,000/year over the last 3 years. Sarah worked as a clerk in the parking and traffic office at the local college until their last child was born. She currently is a homemaker. Ed asked Sarah for a divorce 4 months ago and, although Sarah did not want it initially, she has agreed it is time to terminate the marriage. Ed's lawyer friend suggested that Sarah and Ed use divorce mediation as a method for reaching a divorce settlement agreement. Ed contacted their neighborhood mediation center and made an appointment with a divorce mediator. Sarah has agreed to go to mediation.

THE FIRST SESSION

In their first joint session, the mediator ensured that Ed and Sarah were there voluntarily. The ground rules were explained and they were assured that mediation was confidential because mediators cannot be required to

[1]A composite of individual divorce mediation cases seen at the Cleveland Mediation Center, and reviewed by both authors, was used in this case study.

testify in court and no information from the sessions can be disclosed without the written permission of both parties and the mediator. The only exception to this rule is disclosing facts such as child abuse and or plans to commit a felony, which the mediator is compelled by law to report to authorities.

Because Ed resides in Atlanta and Sarah lives in Ohio, the mediator agreed to schedule three 3-hour appointments on consecutive Saturdays, with the understanding that more time might be needed. The fees will be paid by Ed but they understand that, in fact of law, both Sarah and Ed are paying because the money is really still joint property. They agreed to a fee of $100 an hour.

Ed and Sarah were then told the purpose and limitations of mediation. It was stressed that although a licensed attorney, the mediator is not acting in that capacity. The mediator is also not a counselor, and the purpose of mediation is to make informed decisions about the divorce and the custody of their children. They were urged to consult their individual attorneys at any time during the mediation and before they sign an agreement. Their final written agreement will serve as the basis of their settlement, which they can take to a court of law and have a judge make legally binding.

Ed and Sarah were also informed about the necessity of their full disclosure of assets. They were also reminded that either one of them can withdraw from mediation at any time. They were then asked to each tell what they saw as the key issues that need to be settled and what they would see as an equitable agreement:

Mediator: Ed, would you like to begin?

Ed: Sure. To really understand my position I must first tell you a little about our relationship. We dated for 2 months and married my second year of college. The first 4 years of our life together were idyllic. We were very much in love, we had all the time and money we needed to be with each other and do whatever we wanted.

Sarah: Give me a break! We only had money because I earned it!

Mediator: Sarah, you'll have a chance to explain your side. It's Ed's turn, please try not to interrupt. Go on, Ed.

Ed: Well, what most attracted me to Sarah, besides her uncommon physical beauty, was her strong will and independent nature. She was self-contained, intelligent, and witty. Sarah was not my first girlfriend but I was not terribly experienced with women romantically. I have five sisters and always had as many women friends as I did men friends, but it's safe to say that Sarah was the first great love of my life. As I mentioned, our early married life was like something out of a romantic fairy tale. We had a lot of friends, a great social life, and the freedom to do whatever we wanted. Things began to change after our first child, Ed Jr., was born. In addition to the loss of our freedom, for the first time in our lives we had to budget our money. Because of the expense of child care and increase in my graduate school tuition, our income decreased by a third. We had always equally shared in household duties and I fully expected to share in parenting duties. After the initial euphoria of Ed Jr.'s birth wore off, the reality of the amount of care that was required by an infant set it. We began to argue about who was doing more than the other. I was in my last year of graduate school and really needed to crack the books but Sarah didn't seem to care. All I ever heard was how she was working and I wasn't. So, I started working part time at the local union hall as a bartender. Our income was stable again and I didn't have to work as many hours. We settled into a frenzied but oddly rewarding life of working parents. Our lives were routinized, and a little boring, but secure and comfortable. Things changed dramatically with the birth of our second child, Phil. Sarah announced that she wanted to be a full-time mom and had no intention of returning to work. She claimed her work was unrewarding. We just couldn't afford it. I had just gotten my first job and it didn't pay much so Sarah had to work at least part time. She never forgave me for this. Our relationship had gone from passionate lovers and life partners to petty squabblers, who argued over whose turn it was to take care of our children. The beautiful, intelligent, independent woman I married turned into a slovenly, needy loser who expected me to account for every minute I was away from the house. Our sex life was practically nonexistent, and I pondered the possibilities of an affair. Sarah must have sensed this because within the next year she became pregnant with our third son. She claims it was an accident. She claims that she "forgot" to take her birth control pill. I don't regret the fact that Tom was born. However, had he not been born I would have divorced Sarah years ago. Sarah and I seemed to have reached an understanding soon after Tom's birth. We did not fight the same battles and settled into a comfortable, but by no means loving, relationship. Sarah stopped working and stayed home with the children. I had decided, with the help of my attorney friend, that it was going to be an economic feat of heroism to manage one household on my income, and that a divorce was out of the question for now. I also felt that the boys needed both of us and would especially need me more in a few years, so I decided to wait. Well, the time finally has come. What really triggered this divorce was Sarah's father's death. It was inspiring to witness the love that Sarah and her father had but Sarah's unwillingness to get over his death has ruined us. She cried all the time and accused me of being an insensitive lout who didn't know how to comfort her. The worst of the earlier behavior resurfaced. She resented being "stuck" with the boys but was unwilling to find work. I felt like I was working 60 hours a week, running a household and caring for four children. She gained weight, took no interest in her appearance, and confined her conversation to topics on talk TV shows. I began having a series of "flings" with women I met through work. None were serious and they all understood that I was married and just playing. The closest thing I had to a relationship was with a coworker who was in a similar marital situation. We had an "arrangement" as she called it. I needed to be desired and let myself desire someone. She was transferred and our arrangement is on hold. I don't feel guilty about this because I am too young not to be sexual. However, I value honesty and believe I owe it to Sarah to get out of this marriage. Two months ago I moved to my parents' farm in Georgia. I have lots of business contacts and believe my mother could look after the boys when I'm at work. I think the boys need me and they can visit their mother during the summer. I also want Sarah to get on her feet and I'm willing to give her half the house and the boat as well as 3 months' living expenses. I really just want this thing over.

Mediator: Thank you, Ed. Let me see if I understand what you see as the major issues. First, you would like custody of the boys, you would also like to split the house and give Sarah the boat if she wants it. And you're also willing to give Sarah 3 months' living expenses. Is this correct?

Ed: Yeah, I don't want to hurt Sarah, I just want her to get her life together and get out of mine.

Mediator: OK. We can talk more about that after Sarah has had a chance to tell what she sees as an equitable agreement and the issues she thinks need to be resolved.

Sarah: Well, first of all, I'm having a very hard time with this whole thing. He's a liar, a cheat, ah . . . (mediator interrupts)

Mediator: Excuse me, excuse me, Sarah, I really would like to hear what *you* would like to see happen in this divorce settlement. I'd like you not to focus on Ed but rather on you and what you want. Do you think you can do that?

Sarah: OK, let me start over. To really understand what I want you have to understand what I've done for this marriage. You see, when we first got married, I took my vows very seriously and thought that this thing was a forever deal. Boy, what a fool I was! If I knew then what I know now, I would have never married the jerk.

Mediator: Sarah, try to focus on the future, not the past. Can you tell me about how you see your future after the divorce?

Sarah: Well, yeah, I thought that once Ed got through with school, I'd be able to quit my awful job and stay home with the kids.

Ed: But the kids are in school—what are you going to do all day, sit around and eat ice cream?

Mediator: Ed, it's Sarah's turn to tell what she wants, without interruption. In order to expedite this process we need to abide by the guidelines we agreed to at the beginning of the mediation. You'll both have a chance to discuss the issues once we've had a chance to get them out. Now, let's get back to Sarah. Please continue.

Sarah: I just have to say one thing, then I'll move on—Ed, you are the biggest . . .

Mediator: Please Sarah, just tell us what you want.

Sarah: OK. I feel that because I helped put Ed through college and gave up my 20s to do so, I should be compensated in some way. I not only feel that I gave up career years but also many opportunities to find another mate because look at me now. I'm out of shape from giving him three beautiful children, I'm uneducated and have no future career, I can't find a job, and now he wants a divorce so he can probably be with some bimbo. And *please* don't *bother* denying it!

Mediator: Sarah, remember we are trying to keep this on you, not Ed. So continue. Given the situation you've described, what do you want?

Sarah: I want to be compensated for all my years of dedication and hard work, I want the children, I want the house, I want the money, I want his head on a platter!

Mediator: Sarah, it's clear that you're feeling angry about the past. If you can bring yourself to leave the past for a moment and think about what kind of future you think would be beneficial for you and the children, what do you see? It sounds like Ed and the children love each other, am I right?

Sarah: I don't know why they love him but they do.

Mediator: Well, given that the children love their father, I really don't think you would want to see them suffer.

Sarah: Of course not, I want my children to be happy. And I know he'll have some rights to them but they are *my* children! And he is crazy if he thinks he is moving them to Georgia!

Mediator: OK, Sarah, let me see if I can paraphrase what you've said you wanted. You want to see your children happy. You feel you deserve some monetary compensation for helping Ed through school. You want to stay in the home with the children and be able to maintain your current lifestyle. Is that right?

Sarah: Yeah, I guess. You see, 14 years ago when I took the job as a clerk for the parking and traffic office and gave up the college scholarship money to get married, I really thought that Ed and I were a team and my role was to take care of him and the children and work just to get him through school. I had no idea that someday I'd be sitting here talking about divorce. But I am and I want him to pay for those years.

Mediator: We need to stop for today. From what both of you have said, our agenda for the next sessions should be division of the marital property and the issue of custody, support, and visitation of the children. Is this correct?

Ed: Yeah.

Sarah: Yeah, I guess.

THE SECOND SESSION

There was little disagreement about the worth of the marital property but, as is common, both parties had different ideas for the division of the assets because they had different plans for their lives after marriage:

Mediator: Well, we seem to be off to a good start. We agree on what it is to be divided. Who would like to start by saying what it is they want or what they see as a fair division?

Ed: Well, I have it all worked out. It, of course, depends on Sarah agreeing to a few things. I'd be happy to start.

Mediator: Do you want Ed to go first?

Sarah: Yeah. It's just like him anyway . . . Thinks he always has all the answers.

Mediator: Why don't you go ahead, Ed.

Ed: Well, this is how I see it. We have $120,000 worth of equity in our home. We should sell it and split the money evenly. The boat is only worth $6,000, and there is another $20,000 in our investment portfolio.

Sarah: Are you out of your mind? Where do you expect the boys and I to live? If you think you're going to take $60,000 out of this marriage to chase bimbos, you're nuts.

Mediator: Sarah, it sounds like you have a lot of feelings about this proposal. Before we talk about it, though, we need to hear what you had in mind.

Sarah: What I had in mind? We're sitting here talking about our life together like we're carving up a piece of meat! (long pause)

Mediator: Are there things that you would rather talk about?

Sarah: You're damn right there are! Like how I wasted away my life to make our family comfortable. Like Ed chasing every skirt that came by. Like my giving up my career and chance for a good livelihood. Like me being stuck with no choice in this ending . . .

Ed: I've heard all of this before. That's not why we came here. I'm tired of hearing this poor victim, could have been Madame Curie, crap.

Sarah: How dare you . . .

Mediator: *Whoa!! Stop!!!* Both of you take a deep breath. I don't want anyone to say anything until I say so. (after a couple of minutes) Let's try this again. First, let me say that both of you are going through one of the most stressful events that people face in their lives. It is perfectly normal for people to be emotional and distraught. If people could do this calmly and rationally, they wouldn't need a mediator. Let's try to stay focused on why we are here. Sarah, continue . . .

Sarah: You got the goodies . . . the great career, you kept your looks, you have a social life. I don't even know how I'm going to support myself. I gave it all to you. Or what I thought was us.

Ed: Sarah, you were not a helpless victim in this deal.

Mediator: Look Ed, I'm asking you to listen to what Sarah is saying. You don't have to agree or even like it, but unless you can understand, we'll get nowhere.

Ed: OK. I'm the bad guy, right Sarah? My life has been roses while you suffered. If that what you're saying?

Mediator: Sarah, you have a lot of feelings about the past and you have a right to feel the way you do. You may want to talk to a counselor about these feelings so that you can come to terms with them. But unless we can begin to focus on the future, mediation isn't going to work. Would you like to continue or do you need a break?

Sarah: There are some things that I would really like to clear the air about but I guess now isn't the time.

Mediator: I think it would be best if you told Ed your ideas for the division of the assets.

Sarah: Well, I don't know if you call it division. I want the house, the children, and child support. Because my efforts created the position for Ed to make the big salary, I want a quarter of his earnings until the boys are grown.

Ed: You're a crazy bitch if you think you're getting anywhere near that much.

Mediator: Ed!!! Come on . . . Is that how you talk to anyone?

Ed: I'm sorry. You're right but it's just too much. I'm not going to slave away while she sits in my house in the suburbs.

Mediator: You don't like what you heard. Sarah didn't like your proposal either. At least you have that in common. We're almost out of time so I would like to recap. You both agreed on the property that is to be divided. Ed, you understand that Sarah is feeling afraid and abandoned. Neither of you liked what the other had in mind for the division of assets. Is that accurate? (both nod agreement) OK. I know it doesn't seem like it to you but I actually think we had a good session. What I would like you to do is to think about what you really want. What the other person wants, and what it is you would be willing to give up to get what you want. Are there any questions?

Sarah: I've done extensive research and it seems to me in cases that go to court that infidelity is a factor in a settlement. Is this true and how will we handle that here?

Ed: Give it a rest!!!

Mediator: Sarah, I can't give you a legal opinion. That's why I recommended that you consult your attorney throughout the process. You and Ed will determine what's fair for you.

Sarah: Oh, I have and I will.
Mediator: I'll see you both next week.

THE THIRD SESSION

Mediator: Well, welcome back. You both look rested. Let's pick up where we left off. Let me summarize the initial proposal that you each made. Ed, you suggested selling the house and splitting the revenue generated 50/50. Is that about it?
Ed: Yes, but I want to make a change.
Mediator: I just want to be sure we all understand what has been said. We'll get to new proposals in a minute. Sarah, you said you want the house, the children, child support, and one fourth of Ed's salary until the children are grown. Is that right?
Sarah: Yes but . . .
Mediator: Hold that for a second. I just need to be clear about one other thing. When you said you wanted the house, what did you mean by that?
Sarah: Well, I meant I wanted to stay in the house.
Mediator: Who was going to make the house payments?
Sarah: I wasn't sure. It depends.
Mediator: On what?
Sarah: On how things went!
Mediator: Well, you've had a week to think and consult your advisors. Does anyone want to start the ball rolling?
Ed: I have a few things that I want to say.
Sarah: He started first last time.
Mediator: You're right. Did you want to start?
Sarah: No, I just wanted to point out that he went first last time.
Mediator: What did you want to say, Ed?
Ed: Well, this isn't easy for me to say but I've done a lot of thinking about what was said here last week. Sarah, I don't want you to have to be afraid for your future. I did gain something because you took care of everything else. We were partners and I'm coming out of this in better shape.
Sarah: I think your lawyer told you I was right and infidelity does factor into the settlement! I want it all.
Ed: You know . . . whatever happened or did not happen in my private life has nothing to do with this. If you want to go by what you think the law is and what you have to prove, let's stop this and just go to court. Let's see what you will really get from a judge.
Sarah: Well . . . let me hear your offer.
Ed: You said that you were concerned about your future. You have also made the point that the reason you could not complete your education was that you were a wife and a mother. Here's my offer. I'll take the boys. We'll live on the family farm and Mom will help

with them. We'll sell the house and I'll only take $40,000 and give you $80,000. That way you'll be free of the responsibility of caring for the boys, and have $80,000 to finish your education and become independent.

Sarah: You take the boys? Sell the house? I don't know about any of this. I was prepared to forgo the one fourth of your income but pretty much wanted everything else to be the same.

Ed: You need to get real. You practice a pretty convenient brand of feminism. You blame me, the male oppressor, for denying you your career and when I offer to help you with it, you want to be the dependent Suzy Homemaker!

Sarah: Don't you give me that feminist crap.

Mediator: Let's back up a minute. Calm down, both of you. Can we explore the options that have been presented? Ed, what did you mean when you said you would take the boys? What would be the custody and visitation arrangements?

Sarah: I will never . . .

Mediator: Sarah, you need to hear what it is Ed is offering before you say no. Otherwise we're wasting our time.

Ed: Well . . . my lawyer told me about shared parenting. It means that both parents have the responsibility and say about child-care issues even if the boys stay primarily with one. Visiting would be whenever it could be arranged without being disruptive. No matter what our differences, I would never use the boys to get at Sarah. She has been a good mother and the boys need her in their lives too.

Sarah: They could live with me and I could go to school.

Ed: The money just isn't there. I worked it out. I net $5,000 a month. The mortgage payment is $1,200. Mandated child support is $800. Our household bills, that's your department.

Sarah: $1,800.

Ed: That's $1,200 you want me to live on? We haven't even talked about cars or medical insurance.

Mediator: Ed, are you saying that there isn't enough income to accept Sarah's proposal?

Ed: I'm not only saying it, it's true. Look at the numbers.

Sarah: I don't know about this.

Mediator: You don't believe that there's not enough income?

Sarah: No, I believe that part. I just never pictured not being with the boys.

Ed: You'll be with the boys. They can visit any time you want within reason. They can spend most summers with you.

Sarah: Tell me more about this shared parenting. How would I be involved in these decisions?

Ed: Well, you can decide with me where to send them to school. If there are medical problems, God forbid, we would make joint decisions. We'll decide on braces and anything else that comes up.

Sarah: You know that I want them to go to Catholic schools. You never even go to Mass.

Ed: There are Catholic schools in Georgia.

Sarah: So I'm going to get $80,000. That's a little more than $5,000 a year for all that I did for you. Do you think that's fair? I'm supposed to live on that, pay rent, tuition, and everything else? How long do you think the money will last?

Ed: Come on, Sarah!

Sarah: No, you come on, Ed. I was faithful and alone while you cheated on me and humiliated me. Now I'm supposed to come on?

Mediator: Sarah, can we stick with the issues please? I hear how hurt and angry you are but where is it getting us?

Sarah: I don't know but I just had to say it.

Mediator: Can you tell Ed what you like about his proposal or can you make a counterproposal?

Sarah: Well, I like the shared parenting idea. I guess I'll have to give you the boys for now. I'm just not sure what will happen to me without them. But that's my problem. As far as the rest goes, I'll take $80,000 from the sale of the house and I want you to pay for my tuition through graduate school, I want the investment portfolio, and I want you to pay for a leased car until I graduate.

Ed: This is crazy. Would you tell her to get real?

Mediator: Let's wait a minute here. I think we're getting real close. We have agreement on where the boys will live and unless you were lying, and I don't think you were, the visitation will be liberal and no problem. You've come to agreement on a split for the house. What's left on the table is the investment portfolio, tuition payments, and the lease of a car. No one has mentioned the boat but we have to decide on that also.

Ed: That boat is mine and the investments are for my retirement.

Sarah: Not according to my lawyer.

Mediator: Look, we're real close to settling this. We've been going at it for almost 2 hours. I want us to take a 10-minute break. I'd like each of you to think about these three things: We can come to a settlement within the next 50 minutes and this part of the ordeal will be over. What is your bottom line, what can you live with, and what will you give to get what you need? I don't want you to talk to each other on the break.

After 10 minutes

Mediator: OK, are we ready to finish this? Who would like to start. We have to decide about the boat, investments, tuition, and a leased car.

Ed: This is my bottom line. I'll pay for your tuition through graduate school. You get your own transportation, but I'll pay your medical insurance until you graduate. I get the boat and the portfolio.

Sarah: I'll take the tuition and medical insurance and drop the car. You can keep the boat. I want the investment portfolio for my retirement. That's my bottom line.

Silence for 3 minutes

Ed: You really are something. Here's my last offer. We split the portfolio or everything comes off the table.

Sarah: We split the portfolio but we find a trustee for it. My guy says it's real easy to fool around with those investments. Get one of your bimbos to let you play with her money.

Ed: (long pause) Deal. I want this over.

Mediator: Well, I think that about covers everything. We have an agreement in principle and in some detail about all the issues. The next session will really be a matter of writing it up in a way that will be acceptable to the court. I, of course, want you to review everything with a trusted advisor. Is there anything else?

Sarah: I just want to be clear so you don't think I'm playing games. When I agreed to the living arrangements for the boys, I said for now. I mean until I'm finished with school. I would like to come back here and renegotiate that. Can that be written into an agreement?

Mediator: Sure, if that's what you and Ed agree to. Ed?

Ed: Anything can happen in 3 years. Sure, why not?

Mediator: Well, you both did great work. I'll see you next week to formalize things.

CONCLUSION

The issues raised in this case are typical of couples undergoing a divorce. The goal of mediation is to allow them to design their own settlement and, hopefully, improve their communication with each other. This process differs from traditional adjudication. For example, traditionally the couple's house would be appraised only in terms of its monetary value. Under mediation, however, the financial worth of the house and its sentimental value (if any) are taken into consideration.

As is evident in this case, many of the partners' concerns are emotionally charged and their successful resolution is likely to depend on the skill of the mediator and the willingness of the couple to reach an agreement. It is also evident that power imbalances due to economics, negotiation skill, and knowledge of the law are likely to impact the final outcome. It remains to be seen if mediation, in fact, helps equalize or perpetuate these imbalances.

RELEVANT CONCEPTS

adjudication
conflict resolution
divorce mediation

negotiation
power imbalances

DISCUSSION QUESTIONS

1. Did Sarah and Ed reach a fair and equitable agreement? Why or why not?

2. How were society's attitudes about gender roles reflected in this mediation? Could the gender of the mediator influence the outcome? If so, in what ways?

3. What issues (if any) not mentioned in the final agreement may come back to haunt Ed or Sarah?

4. What were the strengths and weaknesses of the mediator?

5. One of the primary goals of the mediation process is to provide a balance of power between the couple so that a fair agreement can be reached. Describe the power balance between Ed and Sarah (include level of negotiation skill, realistic assessment of economic factors, and other appropriate factors).

6. How might the emotional status of Ed and Sarah affect the outcome of the mediation process?

SUGGESTED READINGS

Cebollero, A., Cruise, K., & Stollak, G. (1986). The long-term effects of divorce: Mothers and children in concurrent support groups. *Journal of Divorce, 10*, 219–228.

Davis, F. (1991). *Moving the mountain*. New York: Simon & Schuster.

Gold, L. (1981). Mediation in the dissolution of marriage. *Arbitration Journal, 36*, 9–13.

Shaffer, M. (1988). Divorce mediation: A feminist perspective. *University of Toronto Faculty of Law Review, 46*, 162–200.

Weitzman, L. J. (1985). *The divorce revolution*. New York: The Free Press.

8 *Elder Care: Different Paths Within an Extended American Family*

Jon F. Nussbaum
Lisa Sparks
University of Oklahoma

Mark Bergstrom
University of Utah

The Oliver family has always been perceived as close and supportive by those who know this family. Louigi Olivieri and his young bride Christina arrived in New York City shortly after the turn of the century. They brought with them three young children and made their way through Ellis Island much like thousands had done before them. The border officials thought Olivieri was not an appropriate American name and officially changed the name to Oliver as Louigi and family were placed on a train to Pittsburgh to join several siblings who had arrived a year before. Louigi had a railroad job waiting in Pittsburgh as well as a very comfortable home that was to be shared with an older brother and his growing family.

Louigi and Christina arrived in Pittsburgh, quickly set up home, witnessed the birth of two additional children, and lived long enough to meet each of their 27 grandchildren. Louigi died first at age 92 in his home with his family at his side. A few years later, Christina died in the same house on a cold winter morning after making sauce for several of her children who were attending Mass. Louigi and Christina never left their home and were constantly surrounded by family members and friends in their Italian-American neighborhood. They lived very long and healthy lives. Louigi and Christina had lived quite well on his railroad pension and had all of their medical needs met by one of their three daughters who had become nurses.

THE CHILDREN

Parents continue to move their families to America for the chance to improve their lives and to give their children the opportunity to have happiness and prosperity unknown to them. Louigi and Christina had accomplished this goal. Their children had all graduated from high school. Those who wished to attend college did and many pursued advanced degrees. Each child raised a family and continued their lives in the greater Pittsburgh area. No child moved more than 30 miles from their original home. The children, however, lived in ways that were very different from the ways of their parents. None of the children died in the various wars of the 20th century, but the additional pressures and bad habits of the century took their toll. The stories of each of these five children are told in the following sections.

Frank

Frank Oliver was the oldest child of Louigi and Christina. Frank moved with his parents to America and attended the public schools. He excelled in school and was sent to college to become a teacher. The smartest students during the 1920s and 1930s were often encouraged to become teachers. Frank became a high school teacher, married, and had two children. Frank showed great promise as a teacher and was quickly promoted to administration. He would end his career as superintendent of one of the large suburban school districts several miles outside of Pittsburgh.

Frank encouraged his children to attend college and each did. Frank's boy was awarded an appointment to West Point. His only son graduated from West Point in the late 1960s, was sent to Vietnam, and was killed in action. Frank and his wife buried their son at the Arlington National Cemetery. Frank's parents never knew the pain of outliving a child. Frank's daughter was also a schoolteacher who had married, bore two children, and moved south. She lived over 1,000 miles away but kept in touch and visited her parents several times a year. Frank retired in the late 1970s, lived on a substantial pension, and traveled quite extensively with his wife. On a warm summer evening, Frank's wife passed away from a cancer in her breast.

As the oldest sibling, Frank received much support from his brother and sisters. He decided to remain in his house and to become active in the neighborhood where he had lived for several decades. As a former teacher, many of his students were living in the community and he rekindled their friendships. Frank volunteered at local hospitals, drove the senior center van, and taught language courses at the community college. In his late 70s, Frank was elected to the city council and continues to fight hard for school funding.

Frank has recently met a very lovely woman who is a few years younger but enjoys traveling, dancing, and the company of a neighborhood hero.

Alice

Alice is the second-born child and oldest daughter of Louigi and Christina. Alice finished high school in the early 1930s, earned her nursing license at a local hospital, and married the son of the local barber. They lived close to home for 10 years, had their first two children, and moved back into the family home when Alice's husband went off to war. Alice lost her husband in North Africa and became the first sibling to become a widow. Alice raised the children in the family home for a number of years until she remarried. Alice married a factory man and moved the family closer to the mills located on the Ohio River. Alice bore four additional children. The children grew, moved away, and Alice lost her second husband shortly after he retired in 1970. Alice did not want to remain in her home, so she sold her home and moved into a Catholic retirement village a few miles east of her home. Alice lived in her own room for a few years but felt lonely and to this day has a female roommate who also is a widow.

The Catholic retirement home was originally located in a rural section of western Pennsylvania. But, as people moved away from the city center, homes quickly surrounded the facility. Alice helped organize a day-care center run by the retirees at the facility, which soon expanded into an adult day-care center as well. Because the great majority of the individuals living in the facility are older widows who live on Social Security and their husbands' pensions from the mills, many have time to volunteer for the day-care centers.

The retirement home has become a focal point for activity within the community. It is not uncommon to have a young child playing at the day-care center, her mother volunteering to serve snacks at the center for the children, the child's grandmother volunteering to help call bingo within the adult day-care center while the great grandmother who actually lives in the center enjoys a game of bingo. Alice has stated many times that she wishes her own children and grandchildren would visit more often, but because they live so far away, she considers all the children and the adults at the center to be her family.

Dominic

Dominic finished high school a year or two after Alice, went to medical school, and served as an Army doctor during the totality of World War II. He was captured by the Germans during the Battle of the Bulge and spent several months as a prisoner of war. Upon his return from the war, Dominic moved into a large house down the street from his family home, married a nurse, and fathered eight children within 11 years. While in the army, Dominic began to smoke several packs of cigarettes a day. This habit continued. Then, at age 57, Dominic suffered his first heart attack. Although told to stop smoking by every physician who attended him and by every member of his family, Dominic continued to smoke.

Dominic had his second heart attack at age 60. At this same time, it was discovered that Dominic had so damaged his lungs that he now needed almost constant oxygen and could no longer see his own patients. Dominic began a 5-year stay at home and was cared for by his loving wife. During this period, Dominic rarely left his home and as each day passed spent more and more time in bed. Dominic's oldest daughter (Christine) had a family of her own and a career as a hospital administrator in Pittsburgh. She often visited and gave her mom a few evenings off each month. Dominic's wife suffered a massive stroke one morning and was rushed to the local hospital where Dominic was once chief of staff. The stroke was severe and quickly took her life.

Immediately following the funeral, all of Dominic's children met to decide how to care for their father. Of the eight children, only two lived in the Pittsburgh area. A decision was made to keep their dad at home. Each of the children would contribute a small amount of money to help with finances while the two local siblings (Christine and Kathy) would do the best they could to keep their dad at home. A nurse was hired to spend the day with their dad and everyone returned to their homes. As a month passed, it became obvious that not only was this arrangement too expensive but their father needed more care. Christine, without consulting her siblings or Dominic, decided to move Dominic from his home to her home. A room that once was the bedroom of a grandchild now became Dominic's room. Christine was now the single care provider for her father.

This arrangement began to cause massive stress within the family. Christine was often gone and felt guilty each time she spent time on the job. Christine's husband was not receiving any attention and their three children had no life at home. The entire family cared as best they could for Dominic, but the family was slowly falling apart. Christine decided her immediate family could no longer tolerate the stress of total care at home. A meeting was called for all the siblings to once again decide what to do with their dad. None of the siblings attended the meeting because they harbored a severe grudge concerning the earlier decision to move their father into Christine's home. Christine decided on her own to place Dominic within a nursing home.

Christine made all the visits to various nursing homes in the area and moved Dominic into a very pleasant nursing home only 2 miles from her home. Money from the sale of Dominic's home would pay for 1 year of care as a private pay patient within the home. After the money ran out, Dominic would have his care payed for by Medicaid. Dominic had a male roommate who suffered a stroke nearly 8 months prior to his admission and could not verbally communicate.

Christine visits Dominic each day after work. She sits down with him for dinner and often reads the evening paper to him. Dominic does not care much for the various activities organized by the nursing home and often intimidates the nursing staff with his knowledge of medicine and proper procedures. Dominic's other children refuse to visit their father and often state how they have been totally left out of his life.

Mary

The fourth child of Louigi and Christina was the first child born within the United States. Mary graduated from high school and attended college during the Second World War. She earned her nursing degree, married a physician, and during the next 10 years gave birth to eight children. Mary left nursing to raise the children, spent the next 25 years caring for her family, and, 2 months after the final child left for college, the physician husband left for a much younger woman. Mary returned to nursing as a private, night nurse for a wealthy steel tycoon who needs constant care.

The children did not react well to the divorce and, though many of the children live close to Mary, prefer to interact with their father while maintaining only minimal contact with Mary. Mary could not afford to remain in the large family home and because her divorce settlement was rather meager, now resides in a small one-bedroom apartment close to downtown Pittsburgh. In addition to the lack of interaction with her own children, Mary has very little interaction with her siblings who regard her divorce not only a sin but a family embarrassment. Mary's nursing duties often require night work, which places an extreme barrier on any social life. Mary talks each day to the postal employee who carries the mail and often will take the bus to the local mall to watch people shop. Mary has had a very difficult time adapting to single life as a women in her 60s with no familial support system.

Martha

Martha is the youngest of the five Oliver children and has just celebrated her 65th birthday. Martha completed her nurse training, married a sales representative (Richard), and raised three children. All three children traveled far from home to attend college and remain with their spouses and children on the West Coast. After working 35 years with the same organization, Richard was forced to retire. Richard did not adjust well to retirement and from time to time feels very depressed. Martha has recently retired from her position within a large medical clinic and hopes to spend much more time with the grandchildren.

The depression Richard feels often results in extended periods of time where Richard remains in the home. Martha does everything she can to comfort and support Richard. Martha, however, has grown increasingly frustrated with Richard's behavior and mood swings. Martha wants to remain active with her friends, travel, do volunteer work, and take more of an active role with her siblings. Richard, however, demands that Martha stay with him in the home. The more time Martha must spend with Richard at home, the more her friends no longer ask her to join them in their many activities. Recently, a number of friends took a bus trip to Atlantic City for the weekend. Martha was not contacted about the trip and now feels rather bad. Martha is having a hard time understanding why her female friends who have lost their husbands are so much more active and happy than she seems to be.

DISCUSSION

The five children of Louigi and Christina each married and had children of their own. The brief description of their lives just presented opens a small window into how this extended family aged during the later part of the 20th century. Two myths of aging become central to their stories. The first myth centers around the notion that all of us will age in quite similar ways. One central component of this myth is the active withdrawal of society from the elderly and the notion that all elderly individuals accept this withdrawal. A real struggle takes place within the lives of those elderly who do not accept a less active role in mainstream society. The lives of the five children provide evidence that not only do we follow different paths of aging but that each of us can, and will if we choose, adapt our own lives in ways to maintain active involvement in society. This adaptation not to be marginalized often becomes an intense struggle against those in society who are uncomfortable with the notion that as we age we do not go gently to the fringes of society. Each of the siblings had triumphs and tragedies. Each of the siblings had different amounts of control over their lives and made choices that helped to determine their unique individual paths of aging.

A second myth of aging that continues to have a significant impact upon our lives is the feeling that our children will become our physical, financial, and emotional support "safety net" as we age, or stated simply, that our children will prevent a disenfranchised elderly class of people. The children of Louigi and Christina stayed close to home and did provide exceptional support for their parents. The grandchildren of Louigi and Christina found themselves in a much more complex, mobile society that presented innumerable barriers to providing similar support for their parents. The decisions faced by adult children today concerning adaptation to new intimate relationships (Frank) or whether or not to place their parent within a nursing home (Dominic) are new to this generation of adult children. The fact that our life expectancy has increased over 20 years in this century has restructured the very nature of the adult-child/elderly-parent relationship. In addition, the role reversal that occurs as adult children become more active in their parents' lives is directly related to loss in the personal control and power of our elderly individuals. This safety net notion is paradoxical. Although it may be true that adult children are available to aid their parents, this help may directly lead to more loss of personal control and to greater disenfranchisement.

We must also not forget that each elderly individual must cope and adapt to a complex interaction of societal and individual changes. From the death of one's child, to forced retirement, to children who move far away, to severe medical complications, those of us who live beyond our 65th birthday will each face numerous life events that will force us to deal with the unexpected, and often unwanted, consequences of long life. Some will choose to remain active in their families and communities, others will decide to disengage from society, whereas others will have no choice as ill health will force withdrawal from mainstream society. The path of long life for each individual will be unique, complex, and always interesting.

RELEVANT CONCEPTS

active versus passive life orientation
adult day care
elderly mental health
institutional care
options for elder care
personal control
social support

DISCUSSION QUESTIONS

1. How did the different ways the children and grandchildren cared for the elderly members of their family act to empower or disenfranchise them?

2. How did the different life events that Frank, Alice, Dominic, Mary, and Martha experienced throughout their lives foster independence or dependence?

3. How does moving into a retirement community impact one's ability to remain an active member of mainstream society?

4. How can a nursing home be more than a warehouse and not marginalize its residents?

5. In what ways can each of the five children of Louigi and Christina remain active, vibrant contributors to their community?

SUGGESTED READINGS

Baltes, M. M., Wahl, H. W., & Reichaert, M. (1991). Institutions and successful aging for the elderly? *Annual Review of Gerontology and Geriatrics, 11*, 311–337.

Knight, B., & Walker, D. L. (1985). Toward a definition of alternatives to institutionalization for the frail and elderly. *The Gerontologist, 25*, 358–363.

Ladd, R. C., & Hannum, C. (1992). Oregon's adult foster care program: A model for community-based long-term care for elderly and disabled. *Community Alternatives, 4*, 171–184.

Nussbaum, J. F. (1993). The communicative impact of institutionalization for the elderly: The admissions process. *Aging and Society, 7*, 237–246.

Zandi, T., & McCormick, N. (1991). Psychological adjustment of elderly women: An ecological model and a comparison of nursing home and community residents. *Journal of Women and Aging, 3*, 3–21.

PART III

ISSUES RELATED TO ABUSE

9 *Responses to Rape: The Contextualization of Violence Against Women*

Sara Alemán
Melissa Lavitt
Arizona State University West

THE INCIDENT

The peacefulness of Sunday morning was always welcomed and treasured. When the week's pace ran at a dizzying speed, the luxury of not using an alarm clock was never taken lightly. Most Sundays began when B decided she had slept enough. She never slept late, but somehow, waking up when she wanted to, as opposed to when work or school demanded it, left her feeling much more rested.

On this Sunday, however, the pounding on the apartment door could not be ignored. The building shook with each blow. The persistent, angry sound would not stop. She hoped someone would call the police, but realized that her neighbors probably would not answer her prayers. B felt she probably knew who was knocking; yet, later, after the event occurred, she felt stunned and shocked. Although the occurrence was not totally unimaginable, this awareness in no way prepared her for dealing with the aftermath of the rape.

As she got up to play out the scene that she sensed was coming, the lock gave out as she reached the door. J was instantly inside; his ranting that had begun outside her door continued. Where was she last night? What was she doing? Who was she with? She heard his interrogation, but not really. B had already begun to "check out." When did she first learn how to do this? She could stand outside herself, observing the scene, almost as if the distance would provide some protection. This time, however, was different. J must have become aware of her ability to turn herself "off" because he was more insistent on breaking through, making certain that B would not tune him out. His whole being was commanding and frightening.

B was suddenly down on the kitchen floor with J on top of her. From her position on the floor, she looked up to her counter, wondering if there was something she could use for a weapon. His weight shifted as he unzipped his pants. B tried rolling out from under J to reach the cabinet with the pots and pans. The large cast-iron skillet would serve her well. It was futile; J pinned her shoulder down hard with the weight of his chest. She was immobile except for her writhing. His weight became more suffocating and the pain more acute as he entered her. J used his forearm to press down on the base of her neck. B was no longer able to speak and she couldn't catch her breath. She began to panic more, fearing she would lose consciousness. The pain that began in the center of her shot down her thighs and legs. His hate intensified with his every movement; B was terrified.

It was so loud in her brain. When would he finish? Why wasn't she able to stop him? If she could remain still, would it be over faster? B mentally went through various possibilities, but she was not able to do much of anything. Her profound fear and humiliation could not distract her from the presence of J and the pain he was inflicting. His smell was intense and foul. He continued his ranting. J cursed her in the most obscene terms, interspersed with terms of endearment. It was sickening. She knew that the best defense was to remain still. Becoming a compliant victim was, she believed, her best strategy to prevent further harm. Anything else seemed to goad him on. She wanted him out of her, off her, and gone; yet, she knew she was ultimately powerless to carry out her wish.

He was done. He was standing over her with a revolting sneer on his face. He casually zipped his pants and left. B remained on the kitchen floor, curled up on her side with her nightgown pulled over her knees and legs. She rocked a while, trying to soothe the pain that still throbbed. She became aware of the morning noises emanating from her neighbors' apartments. Music, ringing phones, and bits of conversation reached her for the first time all morning. She felt so far away from the normalcy of the day.

She didn't know how long she stayed on the floor, or when the crying started. Her whole body felt bruised, stiff, cold, and sore as she got up and headed for the bathroom. An imprint of J was seared into her flesh. B's pores were filled with his smell, her muscles and tissues ached from trying to resist him, and the pain he'd inflicted left a wound deep inside of her. She could not get into the shower fast enough. After she washed and scrubbed, she filled the tub with hot water and emptied the bottle of bubble bath that was kept on the ledge of the tub. She cried until she was exhausted. Her tears mingled with the comforting water. She soaked for a long time uncertain of what to do, if and when she decided to get out of the tub.

The Aftermath

B eventually left the apartment and went to a restaurant, one she had never frequented before. She did not want to run the risk of seeing J. She sat in a booth in the back of the room; she could see who entered before they would be able to spot her, huddled over her tea.

B began generating a list of possible options. She felt she should do something, but was uncertain what form that something should take. That sense of powerlessness lingered. It was a menacing force that threatened to sabotage any goal-directed activity she could envision.

She persevered, working on the list she had begun conceptualizing. B's list included: calling the police, devising a plan of revenge, calling the rape crisis line, moving, or doing nothing. B realized that it would be difficult to figure out what course of action to take when she could not decide if she should tell her friends or her family about the incident with J. In fact, she wasn't sure what exactly had happened. Yes, she was raped, but there were all these details that caused her to doubt her naming of the experience she had endured.

For example, J was not a stranger lurking in an alley; in fact, she was not totally surprised that the rape had occurred. Furthermore, their relationship had been sexual in the past. Does this still "qualify" as a rape? B remembered watching TV movies about women who successfully fought off their rapists. She had been unable to do this and the thought that somehow she could have prevented the attack tormented her.

On the other hand, she thought there were plenty of women who had endured much worse. Plenty. The event got foggier in her mind. Maybe doing nothing was the best idea. Her life was complicated enough. She certainly didn't need this commotion on top of everything else. Yet, she was hurt and angry and tired of feeling put down and, now, vulnerable.

A Feminist Perspective on Rape

A feminist perspective on rape recognizes the political context in which sexual violence occurs and is perpetuated in American culture. From this perspective, sexual violence is the manifestation of societal values that oppress women. Therefore, it is important to recognize that rape is an aggressive and violent expression of men's power. Furthermore, a feminist perspective reminds us that there are societal and cultural messages that explicitly and implicitly sanction the exertion of this power.

Our depiction of the outcome of B's story now examines, in greater detail, aspects of B's life in order to highlight the context in which rape occurs. Because rape is about aggression and power, it is imperative that we examine themes of powerlessness and vulnerability in the lives of women who have been raped. An appreciation of these issues facilitates an understanding of the impact of this tragedy and the meaning that it has in the lives of the women and men.

An understanding of the personal and societal context for this form of sexual violence is particularly important when we recognize that rape is one of the few crimes that requires that the victim "prove" her status as a victim. Quite often, the victim's assertion that she has been raped is called into question. Furthermore, the proof is often affected by characteristics of the victim rather than aspects relative to the commission of the crime. For example, the age, attire, socioeconomic status, and ethnicity of the victim can have an impact on how the crime is responded to by those in the victim's environment. Victims sometimes find themselves in the position of having to defend their innocence in their own attack.

In addition, the nature of the relationship between the victim and perpetrator also has an effect on the eventual outcome of events. Whereas violence (i.e., "battering") is recognized as a possible feature of some domestic relationships, violence that is sexualized (i.e., rape) is frequently overlooked or interpreted as sexual instead of violent. Regardless of the actual facts of the assault, victim and assailant characteristics weigh heavily in the eventual outcome of the case.

Consequently, B's story is very much dependent on who B is and the nature of her relationship to J. Variations in her life situation and history will affect how her story concludes. A feminist perspective becomes most apparent when the circumstances of B's life are examined in terms of what we can learn about the interrelationship of gender, class, ethnicity, and power within society. Not only will the context of the rape affect its outcome for B and for J, but the reader's understanding of these events and characters will also be influenced.

Three versions of B are described with three different outcomes. It is important to note how the event takes on different meanings based on the characteristics and values of those involved, how the response of family, friends, the community, and the legal system is also dependent on the individuals rather than the event itself. Finally, the reader's reactions may be influenced similarly.

OUTCOME #1

Background

Belen is a 27-year-old Mexican-American woman who works as a nurses' aide and attends a community college with the hope of eventually graduating from nursing school. Jose is her husband, from whom she is currently separated. The couple was married when Belen was 18 and discovered that she was pregnant. Because she worked the Saturday night before the rape, her

8-year-old daughter was staying at Belen's mother's house when the attack occurred. Belen has to rely on her mother for baby-sitting when she works at nights. She was very thankful that her little girl did not witness the rape.

The first few years of the marriage were okay, Belen recalls, but things began to get bad when she first decided to go to work; tension increased further when she enrolled in school. Jose grew more and more resentful that Belen was not pregnant and did not seem to want to have another baby. He believed that her career aspirations interfered with his desire for a larger family. Many arguments ensued over these issues. Although things had gotten violent in the past, this was the most extreme form of Jose's aggression.

Response to the Rape

As Belen sat in that restaurant, the thought that stayed with her the most was relief that 8-year-old Alicia was away from home that morning. She had called her mother before they left for church and talked to the cheerful little girl. The sound of her daughter's enthusiasm was still in her ears as she contemplated what course of action to follow.

Because of her work in the hospital, Belen was aware of the rape crisis center. She had seen workers from the center with women brought to the emergency room after a sexual assault. She remembered them as kind, concerned, and helpful. Belen was very aware of the fact that if she wanted her daughter to have a life different from her own then she must make choices that reflected values she wished to instill in Alicia.

Belen called the rape crisis center and talked to one of the volunteers. She described what had taken place and was surprised by the calm tone in her voice. The rape counselor encouraged her to pursue legal action in order to protect herself and her daughter. The potential responses of the police were also discussed. Belen had washed away evidence of the rape and this would adversely affect her case. Furthermore, Jose and Belen were still legally married and a divorce was not something that was likely to occur in the immediate future. Belen began to feel trapped once again by Jose. She could picture his sneer as she felt her options dwindled.

Epilogue

After their phone conversation, Belen agreed to meet the counselor from the rape crisis center at the police station. The counselor knew the female officer who interviewed Belen. An official report was filed and charges were brought against Jose. A description of Jose, along with his address, was given to an officer so that Jose could be arrested.

During Belen's subsequent discussions with the county attorney, however, her desire to seek justice was not as fervent. She initially thought that legal action would send a strong message to Jose so that he would leave

Belen and Alicia alone. The attorney, however, seemed overburdened with more important cases. He kept reminding her that a conviction would adversely affect Jose's future employment.

Eventually, Belen did not follow through on further legal action. The case was dropped, and contact with Jose continued. Although he would threaten her with bodily harm in retaliation for her initial pursuit of legal recourse, he never again raped her. Belen saw Jose until she moved out of town to attend school. It was only after the move that she filed for a divorce. She had no desire to remarry and her status as married, but essentially single, felt comfortable. It was easier to keep men at a distance in this way and to avoid antagonizing Jose.

Belen changed from a carefree person who was able to think about her future with few emotional restraints to a person who began to plan, out of fear, for her eventual escape from her estranged husband. The self-confidence that had grown in the early months of her separation was now gone and her furtive glances revealed a constant fear that she seemed unable to calm. She also began to experience periodic episodes of depression that left her exhausted. She worried that she had lost the battle against those who did not want her to improve herself.

As a result, once she moved out of town, she contacted a local women's group that advertised in the daily newspaper. As she discussed the circumstances that forced her to move to a town without knowing anyone, she began to feel free from the rape. With help she also began to see that she could continue to move forward in her quest for a professional degree, but she would always carry the scars of the rape. She gradually began to regain some of the power that she had lost to her husband and family, who had been unable to understand her needs as well as they understood Jose's.

Belen also realized that her status in her family and community had always been linked to her associations with men. First she had been a daughter, then a wife, and because she had failed to have more children, her role as a mother was evaluated negatively. Therefore, although her wish to have fewer children and vary from cultural norms had caused her pain, she now understood that not following her own direction would, in the long run, cause even greater pain. She decided that in the future her status would be defined by what she had accomplished and not by her association to a man or to her children.

Discussion

Belen's change in status from pregnant teenager to college student to a woman with a future was accompanied by changes in the way power was distributed in her marriage to Jose. The rape was Jose's attempt to "reclaim" what he believed was rightfully his; it was a statement of his need to reassert his power and authority over her. The expression of oppression is clearly evident.

In Mexican-American families it is very important that family secrets remain within the boundaries of the family. By filing a police report, Belen violated this cultural norm. To make matters worse, when she failed to follow through on legal action, she was seen by her family and her community as lacking credibility. Some wondered if she fabricated the story to in order to harm her husband. Her fear of shame and repercussions from her cultural community posed a formidable obstacle that hampered Belen's pursuit of legal action. Yet, it was exactly this ambivalence that brought the indictment against her credibility. Calling the police brought shame, and not following through brought ridicule.

In order to escape the harsh judgments against her from her community, she was forced to leave the area. Although she left because of her loss of face in the community and her family's lack of support, her greatest reason for the departure was, ultimately, the fact that she had been raped. Once she made the decision that she would move, she then saw the benefits of continuing her education without fear and without perpetuating the shame she brought upon her family.

It is sometimes falsely assumed that rape is an unfortunate, but universal, problem. This assumption implies that rape is a tragedy over which we have very little control. In fact, there is evidence to suggest that cultural attributes influence the prevalence of rape. Rape is not an inevitable part of the human condition. Instead, societies that endorse and value male dominance and a disregard for nature have higher rates than those cultures that respect women and feminine values (Griffin, 1981). Hispanic culture, like mainstream American society, sanctions and glorifies male dominance and other expressions of patriarchy.

Belen's case vignette also illustrates the power of naming. Terms such as *marital rape* and *date rape* have only recently become a part of our vernacular. Furthermore, rape has just lately been legally redefined so that marital rape could become legal possibility. With new definitions and revised language, societal perceptions have also been altered, thus paving the way for the possibility of different outcomes for women who have been raped by men with whom they had a relationship. When marital rape became a legal reality, married women could also be offered protection from sexual assault perpetrated by their husbands.

OUTCOME #2

Background

Belinda is a 15-year-old African-American adolescent who lives with her grandmother and 13-year-old brother. Her mother, who has a history of drug problems, sometimes lives with her mother and children as well.

Belinda attempts high school and works part time helping out in the kitchen at a local restaurant. Johnny is her stepfather, who has an off-and-on relationship with Belinda's mother. Johnny will frequently go to Belinda to find out about her mother. He typically asks if her mother has been "using," and whom she has been seeing. Belinda never understood her mother's relationship with Johnny, but vowed that she would never become involved in something so crazy when she grew up.

Johnny began molesting Belinda when she was 11 years old. The molestation stopped when she moved in with her grandmother 2 years ago. In fact, the sexual abuse was one of the reasons why Belinda's grandmother took the children to live with her. Gran and Belinda only talked about the abuse once, but that's all it took to make some significant changes in Belinda's life. It was with great relief that Belinda agreed to move in with her permanently.

Response to the Rape

As Belinda sat in the restaurant, she realized that her grandmother would be returning from church soon. She didn't go because she was still recuperating from a bad cold and Gran thought it best if she took it easy. Time was running out and she needed to decide what she was going to do about the rape.

Belinda adored her grandmother and saw how hard she worked. Unlike her own mother, Gran believed Belinda when she first told her about Johnny doing "nasty" things to her. This morning, however, was more intense; even Gran, who has heard everything, would have a hard time with this one. Belinda guessed Johnny was using drugs again and was not in his right mind. Perhaps he thought her mother was at the apartment, too. Gran never did like Johnny and warned Belinda about how careful she should be around men. Belinda wondered if there were any men that Gran would deem trustworthy. Unlikely.

With these thoughts in mind, Belinda saw the futility in trying to seek justice. She really couldn't picture going to the police with her grandmother and telling them about Johnny. Anyway, child protective services might get involved and she would risk exposing her family to their intrusive involvement. No, Belinda didn't see anyone who could be on her side other than Gran and her brother. Besides, she needed to hurry home.

Epilogue

Belinda never told anyone about the rape. She worried about becoming pregnant or contracting AIDS from Johnny. Gran thought she was "going through a stage" when she noticed how subdued Belinda had become. She eventually got pregnant by her boyfriend and Johnny left her alone.

Belinda's history of sexual victimization was the likely culprit for a number of symptoms that may continue to plague her throughout adulthood. Somatic complaints, such as headaches and digestive problems, became part of Belinda's everyday life. Dissociative episodes also continued. Belinda continued to mentally "go away" during times of stress, and sometimes during sex.

When the baby arrived, she dropped out of school thinking that one day she would get her GED. Her grandmother was upset that Belinda was following the road traveled by so many women in the family and in the neighborhood, but knew that she had been unable to stop Belinda's mother, and now Belinda, from repeating long-standing patterns.

Discussion

There has been extensive research on the long-term effects of sexual abuse on children. Finkelhor (1988) described four categories of trauma that accounted for the various symptoms associated with child sexual abuse. The symptom-producing "traumagenic" dynamics include the following: powerlessness, stigmatization, betrayal, and traumatic sexualization. The dynamic of traumatic sexualization refers to the process by which a child's sexuality "is shaped in developmentally inappropriate and interpersonally dysfunctional ways" (p. 69).

Children who have been molested may grow up feeling "damaged," dirty and different from their peers. Stigmatization describes the way in which the molested child is frequently treated by those around her. Betrayal is obviously felt by the child who was molested by a close family member or friend. She may also feel betrayed by the nonoffending parent who could be perceived by the child as an unreliable source of protection. Finally, children who have been sexually victimized often feel that they are not in charge of their bodies and their lives. The sense of powerlessness pervades other aspects of their lives and may be responsible for the frequency at which they are revictimized.

Wyatt (1990) noted that the dynamics of child sexual abuse parallel the effects of racism, another form of victimization. For example, stereotypes of African Americans, Hispanics, Asians, and Native Americans permeate the media and portray these groups as sexually precocious. The hot-blooded Latin lover is a common stereotype; depiction of African-American men as "sexually charged beasts who desired white women created the myth of the Black rapist" (Collins, 1991, p. 177). The female counterpart to this persona is the African-American prostitute, a common image in popular media.

Betrayal can be a result of the racism experienced by ethnic minority parents as well as by children. The fact is that parents of African-American children cannot protect their children from discrimination and bigotry. Wyatt (1990) noted that ethnic minority children are likely to feel betrayed and disappointed with the realization that their parents are not powerful enough to shield their children from racist encounters with society. This racism is likely to foster a self-image in children of color that they are not as good, smart, or as pretty as their White counterparts. This perception parallels the abused child sense of stigmatization.

Powerlessness is also a likely consequence of racism. When opportunities are blocked, one's sense of hopefulness for the future is impaired. How can a child learn to feel control over her life when employment, education, and housing options are limited? When self-determination is impeded, a sense of powerlessness may ensue.

Thus, for Belinda the rape and years of sexual abuse may have affected her emotional well-being in the same way that her experiences with a racist society adversely affected her. Belinda, like other children of color, often distrusts White authority figures and agencies (i.e., child protective services, police, school personnel). Interactions with the majority culture tend to leave African-American women with a sense of powerlessness, along with the other traumagenic dynamics, that exceeds that of White women due to the marginalization of women of color. Although women, in general, may experience discrimination in our society, women of color are at far greater risk for discriminatory treatment. Therefore, rape victims may decide to stay away from the agencies and institutions of the majority culture. The inability to access safety within the larger White system may intensify feelings of insecurity, inferiority, and self-hate which, in turn, may lead to self-defeating activities on the part of sexual abuse victims.

This case vignette also serves to remind us that sexual violence can occur in many forms and that these can take place throughout the life cycle. The prevalence of sexual abuse of females under 18 (see, e.g., Russell, 1986) may contribute to normalizing sexual violence in adult relationships, whereby the victimized girl is no longer shocked by further episodes of victimization in adulthood. Belinda, by virtue of her gender, class, ethnicity, and unique life circumstances, was victimized many times over.

OUTCOME #3

Background

Betty is a 51-year-old White woman who is divorced and lives alone. She sells real estate and is attending classes to finish her broker's license. Betty is accustomed to being on her own, and, in fact, prefers her solitary lifestyle. She first met Jim at the bar down the street. Betty liked the bar because she was usually left alone. She could enjoy her drink and not be bothered. It felt safe.

The bartender informed Betty that the new guy in the corner was watching her. At first she ignored his presence; she had stopped looking for a "relationship" a long time ago. Betty typically stopped at the bar after work several times a week. She soon realized that Jim was usually there, but she ignored him. As the weeks went by, however, Betty found herself somewhat intrigued by the mysterious stranger. He seemed harmless and sort of attractive.

Approximately a week ago, Betty celebrated the sale of a particularly expensive property. The commission check would be substantial and she planned to splurge when it arrived. She had counted on unwinding with a few drinks at the bar, deciding how she would spend the fruits of all her hard work.

After a few drinks she was feeling pretty good and a little more gregarious than was typical for her. With only minimal encouragement from the bartender, she sent a drink over to Jim's table. Although she usually avoided his gaze, this time she turned and smiled at him when he lifted his glass in thanks. With a welcome from Betty, Jim joined her at the bar.

Jim continued to stare at her. Conversation was awkward, which Betty attributed to Jim's shyness and the fact that she was feeling the effects of the alcohol. Jim said he was new in town and asked her about places to live. Betty could sound like a realtor regardless of the number of drinks she had! She also told him about a vacancy in her building which was in a nice area of the city—near shopping and the transit system. In fact, she wrote down the address of her building along with a few other rental prospects.

She pretended not to notice when he rested his hand on her arm. When he began massaging her shoulder and neck, she looked him straight in the eye as if to say, "I know what you're doing and I'm deciding what I want to do about it." Twenty-five years ago she might have risked being picked up by a stranger. Older and wiser, she now knew better.

As Betty got up to leave, Jim volunteered to walk her to her car. "You can't be too careful," he warned. At the car, he suddenly grabbed her and brusquely attempted to kiss her. Betty, who usually thought she was a pretty good judge of character, was taken by surprise and frightened by Jim's actions. She got in her car and drove off. She decided not to return to the bar in order to avoid another encounter with Jim. Although she stayed away for over a week, Jim found her that Sunday morning.

Response to the Rape

As Betty sat in the restaurant, she realized with anger how long it had been since she felt this afraid. She hated Jim for taking away the sense of security she had. She needed to do something with her anger, she reasoned.

Thoughts of ignoring the incident were replaced by a growing sense of rage. She called her friend who worked as a paralegal. She couldn't imagine calling the police and describing how foolish she had been in the bar last week. She felt her friend, who was familiar with the legal system, could best help her through the process. Her friend met her at the restaurant and they contacted the police together.

Epilogue

Betty pressed charges and endured the lengthy legal proceedings. Eventually, Jim plea bargained and received minimal jail time. Although the nightmares and insomnia gradually subsided, nights continued to be difficult for her. Noises in the apartment or outside would keep her awake for hours. Although she had vowed she would never own a weapon, Betty bought a gun soon after the incident. She never returned to the neighborhood bar.

Approximately 6 months after the rape, Betty realized that the more acute symptoms, such as her fearfulness, had subsided. She was left, however, with a pervasive and gnawing sense of melancholy. She no longer derived pleasure from her job, her friends, and her other activities with the same consistency and intensity that had existed before the rape. She tired quickly and she began to feel old. In fact, she told her doctor during her check-up that "middle-age had finally arrived." What the doctor and Betty did not realize, however, was that Betty exhibited classic signs of a mild depression.

Discussion

Eighty percent to 90% of rapes are committed by a person known to the victim, with the most likely assailant being a current or former male partner (Allgeier, 1987). Sexual assault committed by a stranger is less likely to occur in spite of its prevalence in movies and on television.

The media would also lead us to believe that rape is a spontaneous act, possibly instigated by the way a woman is dressed, how she behaves, or how much she has had to drink. In reality, however, rape occurs with a great deal of forethought. Ninety percent of rapes are planned in advance and without knowledge of how the victim will dress (Scully, cited in Wood, 1994). The sexual assault is not a reflection of the woman's irresistibility. Instead, it is an expression of aggressive and sexualized force that can occur within a relationship.

Because the victim is very likely to know or be familiar with her attacker, filing a report has implications for the relationship that many women wish to avoid. Thus, the majority of rapes are unreported. The decision not to report intensifies a woman's sense of helplessness and loss of control over her own life, body, and safety. Betty is the exception because she chose to follow through with filing charges. In spite of her willingness to access available resources, however, she was not protected from experiencing symptoms as a result of the rape.

The physical and psychological consequences of sexual assault vary according to the individual, the circumstances of her attack, and the passage of time. The immediate psychological consequences typically differ from symptoms experienced months after the assault. For example, intense fear, shock, numbness, confusion, and extreme helplessness may occur right after the rape. Many of these symptoms relate to women's fear that the attacker will return. It has been reported that symptoms begin to subside by the third month; however, 25% of rape victims will experience severe and long-term symptoms (Hanson, 1990). Furthermore, symptoms that have diminished may later reappear if something in the environment acts as a trigger to psychologically "remind" the victim of her attack. The most common psychological repercussions of rape include anxiety, depression, sexual dysfunction, substance abuse, and posttraumatic stress disorder. Thus, the experience of victimization does not necessarily end when the attack is over.

QUESTIONS AND COMMENTARY

Is the Prevention of Rape Possible?

Some feminists have argued that the prevention of rape is only possible if we effect some fundamental changes in society. This is a radically different approach from most research and social programs on rape prevention. Instead, most prevention programs typically focus on controlling women's activities in order to protect us. For example, educating women about personal safety and advising them to avoid places or situations that may pose a potential risk are features of a typical rape prevention program. Other rape prevention efforts have focused on controlling the offender either through incarceration and stiffer sentencing, or through rehabilitation to "cure" him.

Sparks and Bar On (1985) argued that sexual violence against women is endemic in our society. They suggested that, "We need a social order in which men do not learn to be sexually violent toward women" (p. 2). Sexual violence can only be prevented if we eliminate those conditions in society that perpetuate and encourage its existence. Prevention, therefore, is reconceptualized. The goal of prevention is not merely protection from victimization, but an overall decrease in the likelihood of sexual violence ever occurring in our society. In this light, rape prevention is not similar to crime prevention. Instead, it becomes part of a larger movement for social justice. This movement should ideally reject the notion that violence is inevitable and, therefore, normal. Insistence that women's safety becomes a priority on the public agenda could counteract the tacit acceptance of sexualized violence. Political action, community organization, and education for both men and women could conceivably be part of a true rape prevention program.

What Is the Connection Between Politics and Rape?

The political context of violence is often overlooked or totally ignored. Yet in order to understand violence, its prevention, and an appropriate response to it, the event must be contextualized. The violence must be examined and understood with an appreciation and awareness of the history and current predicaments of the individuals and larger systems involved. Violent acts are often approached as if the event occurred in a vacuum, or as if the context were devoid of racism, sexism, and other forms of discrimination. Feminists have suggested, however, that all events are contextualized in race, gender, and class. Rape is no exception. As we have noted, the gender, race, and ethnicity of the victim, the perpetrator, and even the investigating personnel are part of the context of this crime. How a victim is treated by medical, legal, and counseling personnel may be dramatically influenced by how similar or dissimilar the victim and service provider are. For example, the type of treatment received by a White victim of a White perpetrator may be significantly different from the treatment received by a White victim of an African-American perpetrator. The total experience is contextualized in a political arena that has a long-standing history of racism, discrimination, and sexism.

Other factors that influence the politics of rape include the nature and accessibility of resources that are available to women who have been victimized. Resources are more likely to be accessible and, in fact, utilized if they are located in or close to ethnic communities and staffed by women of diverse ethnicities. If the woman, who has just been violated by a man, has to speak to a man on the other end of the phone to report the event, what are the chances that she will actually file a report? If the emergency room personnel are all White and the victim is African American, Latina, or Asian American, will they be able to comprehend the cultural significance of the attack? We suggest that in most cases the resources and services that a rape victim may encounter are, in fact, affected by racial or ethnic issues. Issues of race, ethnicity, and social class are political in the sense that they play a role in the distribution of resources and power in our society.

If all the players were colorblind, all victims would be treated the same. Victims are first assessed through color-sensitive lenses and subsequent procedures reflect how the color was seen and interpreted. Thus, victims may be further victimized by discrimination based on skin color and/or socioeconomic status. This discrimination may result in limited access to the benefits that our society has to offer in the legal, medical, or psychological field. Differential access and the use of power-enhancing societal institutions is ultimately a political issue.

Why Would Someone Not Report a Rape?

Women are typically not afraid to report a violation of their property. Yet, they are reluctant to report violation of a more personal and devastating nature. The strongest prohibition against reporting a rape is fear of retaliation. The act of rape signifies such abject humiliation and helplessness that women often perceive themselves as lacking in strength sufficient to take on the rapist in any arena. Thus, they remain silent, inadvertently offering protection to their assailant.

This sense of helplessness and shame is often reinforced by societal institutions such as courts and hospitals. This public forum of police, lawyers, judges, and physicians, supposedly there to assist victims, can be severely limited in its ability to reach out to victims because of its adherence to policies that have been, historically, imbedded in a male-dominated political arena. What this means is that all policies related to sexual violence were created in an environment that dictated that sex not be a topic for public consideration and discussion. Furthermore, traditional thinking often tacitly condoned men's violence against women. Thus, traditional thinking has stressed the sexual aspects of rape, and therefore, placed a violent act on a par with an acceptable private and consensual activity.

If rape is to be accurately perceived, then this dual identity of sexualized violence must be reexamined and the presence of force or coercion, rather than mutual consent, must be highlighted. If a crime has been alleged, then the American system requires that someone be held accountable. Quite often, the responsibility has been very conveniently placed on the female with the questions such as "What was she wearing?," "Was she a virgin?," "Did she invite him into her apartment?," and so on. In other words, the emphasis was on treating the victim as the perpetrator and holding her accountable for making herself so *inviting* that the man had no choice but to act according to some genetically prescribed behavioral imprint. If the man were to be "blamed," then it would follow that a crime had, indeed, been committed. Because rape and sexual assault do not "look" like typical acts of aggression in the eyes of men and legal institutions, the criminal aspects of the act are often overlooked. After all, women have historically been charged with the task of controlling or "civilizing" the impulses of men. Therefore, what occurs sometimes is that a victim is reluctant to trust a system that blames her for her victimization.

Although this is certainly applicable within the majority culture, it may even be more prevalent within ethnic cultural groups. As we have noted, women must deal with the significance of violence against women within their own culture. Thus, another reason why women may not report a rape is because skin color and the anticipation of racism may limit their options. For example, many African-American women fear that reporting an African-American man for raping her may, in fact, be tantamount to a death sentence for him. Her fear of her African-American assailant is not as great as the fear of a judicial system that has historically practiced racism. When the system that purports to protect everyone is found lacking, it is less likely to be utilized. Many policies and procedures reflect the values and world view of the majority culture and may not adequately serve the needs of ethnic groups. The array of services that may be available to victims is based on what White society determines victims' needs to be.

In conclusion, American society, and the legal system in particular, may inadvertently intensify the trauma of rape by looking for reasons why the event occurred. Cause-and-effect thinking and the assignment of blame are very much a part of our country's system of justice. It is our contention that linear cause–effect reasoning is not illustrative of a feminist perspective. A feminist perspective, with its emphasis on context, sees rape as a logical manifestation of prevailing social and cultural values. We are bombarded by images that depict women as potential victims. The "sexier" they appear, according to culturally endorsed standards of attractiveness, the likelier it is that they are victimized in our movies, music videos, and advertising. Men, on the other hand, are not only the probable perpetrators, but are also depicted as being preoccupied with sex. Both genders are limited by these stereotypes. A feminist perspective requires that all of our culturally sanctioned stereotypes be reexamined and lifted so that neither gender is victimized and White majority culture is not the sole recipient of societal privilege. It is not a matter of merely holding one individual culpable for the commission of rape. Instead, it is argued that societal values, as reflected in our laws, policies, and institutions, are responsible for perpetuating and tolerating sexual violence.

RELEVANT CONCEPTS

consent versus coercion
contextualization of rape
feminist perspective of rape

patriarchy
traumagenic dynamics
victimization

DISCUSSION QUESTIONS

1. How do you compare your reactions to the "faceless" account of the rape to your reactions when the identities of the victim and perpetrator were revealed?

2. What do the myths about rape say about our society's conceptualization of the problem of rape? How do these myths and misperceptions perpetuate the problem?

3. What is meant by "the personal is political"?

4. What is the difference between rape prevention and intervention?

5. How would you design a rape awareness program? How would this design differ for various audiences?

REFERENCES/SUGGESTED READINGS

Allgeier, E. R. (1987). Coercive versus consensual sexual interactions. In V. P. Makosky (Ed.), *The G. Stanley Hall lecture series* (Vol. 7, pp. 7–63). Washington, DC: American Psychological Association.

Collins, P. H. (1991). *Black feminist thought.* New York: Routledge, Chapman & Hall.

Finkelhor, D. (1988). The trauma of child sexual abuse: Two models. In G. E. Wyatt & G. J. Powell (Eds.), *The lasting effects of child sexual abuse* (pp. 61–82). Newbury Park, CA: Sage.

Griffin, S. (1981). *Pornography and silence: Culture's revenge against nature.* New York: Harper & Row.

Hanson, R. K. (1990). The psychological impact of sexual assault on women and children: A review. *Annals of Sex Research, 3*, 187–232.

Russell, D. E. H. (1986). *The secret trauma: Incest in the lives of girls and women.* New York: Basic Books.

Sparks, C. H., & Bar On, B. (1985). A social change approach to the prevention of sexual violence toward women. *Work in Progress, 6*, 1–8.

Wood, J. T. (1994). *Gendered lives: Communication, gender, and culture.* Belmont, CA: Wadsworth.

Wyatt, G. E. (1990). Sexual abuse of ethnic minority children: Identifying dimensions of victimization. *Professional Psychology: Research and Practice, 21*(5), 338–343.

10 *When the Protector Is the Abuser: Effects of Incest on Adult Survivors*[1]

Eileen Berlin Ray
Cleveland State University

> *I remember the first time he raped me. I was about 7. He thought I was sleeping but I wasn't. He laid down on the bed beside me, lifted up my nightie, and . . .*

THE SETTING

It is a day-long retreat for adult survivors of incest. There are 22 women there, at varying stages of recovery. Some are White, some are persons of color. Some are in their 40s and 50s, some are in their 30s, some are in their 20s. Some are white-collar professionals, some are blue collar, some are unemployed. Some are straight, some are bisexual, some are gay. Some have battled addictions to alcohol and drugs, some never have. Some have been in therapy for years, some have just begun therapy, some have refused therapy altogether. Some were abused by their fathers, some by their step-fathers, some by their mother, some by a grandfather, some by an uncle, some by a brother, and some by a combination of relatives. Some had never told anyone until they were adults, some had told when they were children. Some have confronted their perpetrator and family, some plan

[1]This case is a composite drawn from extant literature and interviews with adult incest survivors. I thank these women for their willingness to share their stories with me.

to, some swear they never will. Some know they weren't responsible for their incest, some aren't sure, and some are certain it was all their fault.

Each of these women has her own story and each of their stories is poignant. They are difficult to hear, to write about, and to read. These women do not speak in unison. Each of them has been impacted by her abuse to different extents and in different ways and each woman has chosen to deal with her incest in her own way. But these differences are irrelevant. It is what they share that brings them together, that transcends their differences. All had been sexually molested by a relative when they were children. Their experiences, their coping, their struggles, and their resilience are evident in their words.

The Retreat

After their introduction, the two facilitators, Rachel and Leigh, explained that the goal of the retreat was to give the women a safe place to talk about their incest and its impact on their lives and to get support from each other. The women were assured that no one would be forced to participate; they could share as much or as little as each woman chose. However, virtually all of the women had come to the retreat planning to participate to the extent each felt comfortable. After explaining that everything said at the retreat was confidential, Rachel and Leigh opened it up to the group.

Karen began, "I remember the first time he ever touched me, just like it was yesterday. I was 9 at the time, an only child. I was very studious and serious, probably because things at home were a mess. My father was an alcoholic and my mother took a lot of prescription medications, like Valium, so she was out of it quite a lot. But back in those days, it wasn't uncommon for women to be put on those drugs so that they'd stay compliant. Anyway, she didn't work outside the home but she had these two women friends and they got together every Wednesday night, no matter what, for dinner and maybe a movie. Most of the time, my dad would go out as soon as she left and leave me with a neighbor. The neighbor, Donna, was about 32 and divorced and she seemed to like having me over. So I felt OK about that. It was better than sitting at home watching my dad get drunker and drunker until he passed out."

"Anyway, one Wednesday night, he didn't leave after Mom did. I was sitting on the sofa watching TV. Occasionally he had slapped me around but that was about it. This night, he had had a few beers but I wouldn't say he was drunk, maybe just a bit tipsy. He came over and sat down next to me and put his arm around my shoulder. I could smell the beer on his breath and it made me feel sick so I pulled away. He didn't like that. He grabbed my arm and said, 'Don't you ever pull away from your father. You're mine and don't you forget it.' He seemed really mad and I was scared so I just nodded. He put his arm around my shoulder again. I just sat there, staring at the TV, stiff as I could be. After a little while, his hand dropped to my chest. On reflex, I pulled back. He got really mad and pushed me down on the sofa. He slapped me and said, 'You bitch, I told you to never pull away from me. Now look what I'm going to have to do to you.' That's when he raped me. I remember the beginning but that's all. I completely dissociated. After he was done, he said, 'Remember, you're mine and this is between us. If you ever tell anyone, and I mean *ever*, I'll kill you.' Then he went into the kitchen and drank until he passed out. When I could finally move, I was shaking and there was blood on the sofa. I tried to clean it up as best I could. I felt numb and scared, petrified. I climbed into bed and huddled under the sheets and cried myself to sleep."

Karen had told her story as though she was a reporter. There was no emotion, just the "facts." But many of the women were now crying, obviously moved by her story. Beth went over and tried to take Karen's hand. Karen smiled and said, "It's OK. I'm fine." So Beth let go and just sat there.

"My mother was a nurse and she worked different shifts. My dad was a carpenter so he was home sometimes during the day and almost always at night," Mary said. "I remember when I was real little, like 4 or 5, and he'd be there while she was at work. He'd give me a bath and act like he was washing me. But then he'd put his hands and fingers in the wrong places. All the time, he'd be talking sweetly to me, saying what an angel I was and how much he loved me and how he was so pleased that we had this special secret that we must never tell anyone or he would have to leave the family and I wouldn't have a daddy anymore. Then he'd dry me off and . . . I'm sorry, I just can't say it." Someone handed Mary a box of Kleenex as she tried to stop her sobs. She pulled her knees up to her chest and started rocking back and forth.

"My mother worked nights, so when she was gone, my stepfather would force me into their bedroom and rape me, orally and vaginally," Carla said. "It started, as best I can remember, when I was about 6. I didn't know what he was doing, just that it hurt a lot. At first I'd always cry but then he'd slap me and tell me that if I wasn't quiet, he'd tell Mom and then she'd know what a filthy animal I was. Little did I realize he never would have told her. But I was scared to death, in terror. He kept doing it until I got my period. I guess he got worried about getting me pregnant. To this day, my sex life is lousy. I usually dissociate and get no pleasure out of being with anyone, man or woman. My mom's still married to him. I've never confronted him or told her. She really loves him. I don't think she'd believe me."

"Boy, do I know what you mean about sex. I can't have sex unless there are all these ground rules. Like the lights have to be on, he can never approach me from behind, like to put his arms around me, and he has to talk to me the whole time. I have to keep hearing his voice. Otherwise I flash back to my stepfather. He'd come in when it was dark and always sneak up from behind and he never said a word. And I have to change the sheets as soon as we're done because I can't stand the smell. It just brings it all back and I start seeing it all again and I start screaming. I'm lucky I have such an understanding husband," commented Lucy. "And, yeah, I didn't think my mother would believe me either. But after I had been in therapy for about 2 years, I finally decided that she needed to know. Well, actually, *I* needed for her to know. It got to the point where not telling her meant I was still keeping the secret and that wasn't helping me. And while part of me didn't expect her to believe me, some part of me really hoped she would. So after rehearsing what I was going to say to her with my therapist, I called her and said I needed to talk to her about something privately. We set up a time and she came to my apartment. Then I told her. And I was right, she didn't believe me. She got real defensive and said I was just trying to upset her and that Jim would never have done those things to me. Somehow I stayed very calm and kept repeating that it didn't matter if she believed me or not, I knew it was true, and it wasn't a secret anymore. She kept trying to argue but I refused to. So after a while, she got up to leave and said for me not to contact her until I had come to my senses. That was about 7 months ago and we still haven't talked to each other."

"I was lucky," said Sharon. "When I told my mom what my dad and brother had done to me, she was shocked. But her first words were, I believe you, I love you, and I am so sorry. She held me for a real long time. Both of us were sobbing. We talked and talked about it and she asked if she could see my therapist with me. So we've done that a few times and it helped. Just knowing she believes me made a huge difference. That night we confronted my dad. They didn't have a great marriage to begin with. He didn't deny it but he said I was making a big deal out of nothing. She threw him out of the house. My brother doesn't live at home so a couple of days later we went to his apartment. He said he never touched me and that I was a liar but she stuck by me and told him to never set foot in her house again until he was ready to deal with the truth. Now she's divorced my dad and my brother still hasn't shown up. She's in a lot of pain but she's seeing a therapist and that seems to be helping. It's incredible; the effects go way beyond the abused child."

Jenny spoke. "That's incredible. What a mother you have! I told my mom about what my brother and my cousins did to me. How they pulled me into the field behind our house, tied my hands behind my back, stuck a rag in my mouth, and took turns raping me. She said I was crazy and a liar and I was just imagining things. That they would never do such a horrendous thing and she never wanted to hear about it again. I told my father, they're divorced, and he said, 'Well, maybe it did happen, but you know, boys can be pretty wild sometimes.' I felt like jumping off a bridge. I still do sometimes."

"My folks said the same kinds of things when I told them about my uncle," said Lisa. "He's my dad's brother. He lived with us for a couple of years when he was out of work. I was about 9, I guess. I can't even talk about what he did to me and what he made me do to him. But I told my parents in general what happened. My dad defended him and told me I must have led him on. My mom asked why I found it necessary to dredge up the past. I was an adult now and I should just let bygones be bygones. Whatever respect I had for them went right out the window. What they said makes me furious. But it's not like they're the only ones."

"Yeah, the last thing my parents want to do is deal with it." Terry spoke up for the first time. "I mean, how can my mother live with herself if she acknowledges that she might have been able to stop it. I don't know if she could have or not. She was scared to death of him and he'd beat her sometimes. But I knew she could hear my muffled screams. I was only two doors away from her room. I was only 10 when it started. She must have known. But maybe it was what she had to do to survive. She didn't have any skills, no money, she was completely dependent on my dad. There weren't battered women's shelters then. Part of me can understand why she did what she did but part of me feels such a deep rage towards her, deeper than what I feel towards my father. She refuses to talk about it, won't even acknowledge it. I could never put my husband ahead of my children. He can defend himself, but my kids are defenseless. Hell, our job as parents is to protect our children."

"Yeah, to protect them and to make sure they like themselves," commented Anne. "You know, I have a job with a lot of authority. I'm responsible for a large budget, I have 13 people working for me. Everybody thinks I'm upbeat and very competent. But they don't know the real me. The only people who know are my two best women friends and my therapist. I feel like a fraud. I know how low a person I am because I know what he did to me. If I was a decent person, he never would have done it."

Immediately several group members got vocal. "Hold on," said Gina. "It had nothing to do with you. You were there, that's it. It was all his fault. You did absolutely nothing wrong and there was, and is, nothing wrong with you."

Marsha immediately echoed Gina. "I felt like you do for a long, long time. I mean, my father told me that I was a slut and that no man would ever want me if he ever found out what I did. I could never get close to a man. Sex was fine, that's all I figured I was good for. But a real relationship was out of the question. If it was a real relationship, then I'd have to tell him about the incest and then he'd get rid of me. I believed my father. It has taken me years of therapy to finally really believe that my father is a very sick man and what he did was inexcusable and that it wasn't my fault. But it's been a long road getting to this point."

"Well, maybe it wasn't your fault but I know for a fact that it was me who caused it to happen," argued Sandra. "It's different for me. It was my grandfather. I sought him out, I let him do it. I gave myself to him. And even though I knew it was wrong, it felt good and he never forced me and I didn't try stop him."

"Hold on, Sandra." Peggy stepped in. "Of course it might have felt good. He knew just what he was doing. He's an adult, he knows what to do, where to touch you, so that your body responds. He set you up so that he wouldn't have to force you and so that you'd want to come back. Tell me, what were things like in your house?"

"Well," Sandra said, "things weren't very good. My sister and brother are much older than me so they were out of the house by the time I was 8. My father worked all the time so I didn't see him very much. When he was home on weekends, he was usually out with friends. I don't remember having more than a couple of conversations with him. He'd say hi and ask how I was and then be on his way. My mom didn't work but she was always gone, I'm not sure doing what. She'd leave notes around the house saying I had to do my homework, start dinner, vacuum, sort laundry, that kind of thing. They didn't like me to have friends over, and I really didn't have many friends. I was pretty lonely and watched a lot of TV."

"And what about your relationship with your grandfather before he started molesting you?" asked Lucy.

"From as early as I can remember, I adored him. He thought I could do no wrong and we were always very affectionate, very huggy. And my parents encouraged that, always saying how wonderful it was that I had such a special relationship with him. He called me his sweetheart and I always felt special when I was with him."

"Can you see," said Jenny, "how he was giving you everything your parents weren't? He knew where you were vulnerable and stepped in. I'm not saying he meant to hurt you. He may have really loved you. But he was a sick man and what he did to you he did because he knew you were so starved for love, that he had a prime target. It's not your fault that your parents ignored you or that you responded to his attention and affection. That's what kids need and crave."

"Well, I'd never thought about it that way before." Sandra had tears streaming down her face. "I mean, the incest is bad enough but I guess I'd always believed in a strange way that at least he thought I was special.

I mean, that's what he always said whenever he was doing it. That I was the most special person in the world to him, that he loved me so much. Now you're saying that those were just empty words, he just wanted a child's body, any child's body, and I was compliant. It's kind of like a guy using all the right lines to get a girl into bed. She falls for them, trusts him, sleeps with him, and then he's gone."

"I know exactly what you mean, Sandra." DeAnne spoke up. "I still blame myself. In my head I know it wasn't my fault, that I was only a child, all of that makes sense. But in my heart, I don't believe it. Why didn't I do something? Why didn't I scream or kick him or fight him?" I must have wanted it. I mean, there were other people in the house. If I had made noise, they would have heard me. And I hate myself for not trying to stop him. At least then, even if it hadn't worked, I could feel like I had at least tried to stop him."

"But DeAnne," said Carla, "what really might have happened if you had tried fighting back? He might have gotten really angry and taken it out on you. And what kinds of things did he say to you?"

"He said that if I ever told anyone, he'd beat me up so bad that I'd wish he had killed me. Pretty nice guy for a father, huh?"

"What a bastard! Well, I sure wouldn't want to risk that," said Mary. "Any kid would be petrified to hear her father say that. You're looking at it as an adult looking back, so it's pretty easy to be rational and powerful. But remember back to how you felt as a child, when it was going on. Not only were you physically much smaller, you were dependent on this pervert for your life. That's the thing, the people you're supposed to be able to trust are the ones who are abusing you. If it was someone outside the family, they'd be the ones you'd go to for help. But it's them, so you have nowhere to go and no one to trust. It's amazing any of us have put together any kind of workable life."

"Yeah," said Kate. "When I look at my life now, I'm pretty amazed. I've done a lot of drugs and spent a lot of time drunk. And I tried to kill myself twice. I almost did it, and at the time I was miserable that I had failed at that too. The pain doesn't just end because he stops abusing you or because you grow up. The damage that's done gets into every part of your life, every relationship you have. I can't keep a man, I can't keep a job. My ex has the kids and I only get to see them once in a while but it's better that way. I'm too screwed up to do them much good. In some ways I'm better now than I've ever been but I still have trouble keeping it together and there are still times when I wish I was dead. It's just so hard and it hurts so much." Tears were freely flowing down her face. Karen, sitting next to her, took her hand.

"I tried to kill myself too, about 10 years ago," added Lisa. "I got into the bathtub, filled it with some hot water, and slit my wrists. I watched the blood coming out and I started to feel dizzy. I felt like I was floating. It was the best I had felt in a long time. I thought I had finally found the peace I was looking for. I guess I passed out because the next thing I knew, I was in an ambulance on the way to the hospital. My roommate had unexpectedly gotten off work early and came home so she found me. I spent a few months on a psychiatric unit and got on antidepressants. That's helped some but I know what you mean, Kate. I still see killing myself as an option. But I've got my daughter living with me. That's the only thing that keeps me going."

Sitting over in the corner, Carol was curled up crying. Leigh gently asked, "Carol, can we help? Do you want to talk about it?"

"One night, when I was about 8," Carol began, "I remember waking up in the night feeling scared. I went to my parents' bed and climbed in with them. I was lying on the outside, next to my mother. She woke up, saw it was me, and asked why I was there. I told her and she said I could stay. The next thing I knew, she had her arms around me, holding me very close. It felt good in some ways but it was kind of hard to breathe. But then I felt one of her hands go down to my private parts and she started messing around with me. It hurt a lot. I laid there as still as I could, trying not to breathe. Once I was sure she was asleep, I got up to go back to my bed and saw a little bit of blood on the sheet. I didn't know exactly what had happened but I knew I was shaking and crying. After that, I would never let myself be alone with her if I could help it. And if she tried to comfort me, I pulled away. We never spoke about it and I never told my dad. He's dead now and I never see her. But I remember it as if it were right now."

No one said a word. Everyone else in the group had been molested by men. They had never even considered that the perpetrator might be the child's own mother. They were horrified and stunned. Several people had tears streaming down their faces and someone put her arm around Carol, who was sobbing.

"I don't know what to say," offered Julie. "Why would the people who are supposed to love us, the people we're supposed to trust, do these things to us?" People shook their heads, wishing they had an answer but having none.

"We have to remember that they're the ones responsible for their perverted behavior, not us. They tried to make us think it was us forcing them to abuse us, but that's just bull. But what really makes me mad is that we have to pay twice. First, when we're being abused as kids and now again as adults. And in many cases, the perpetrator gets off and is never held accountable for all the damage he's caused," Lucy said angrily.

"Boy, you hit the nail on the head," Denise said. "In some ways this is worse than the actual abuse because this time I *know* what's happening and I have the feelings with it. Then I just dissociated; I don't remember feeling anything. That helped then but it sure makes getting any work done or taking care of the kids or driving the car harder. I'm furious that what he did to me is invading my life now."

"I confronted my stepfather and told him that I was going to tell my mom and all his family and friends. He got really scared and said he'd do whatever I wanted him to do but he begged me not to tell Mom or anyone else. I told him I'd think about it but that he had to pay for my private therapy. He has a good job and enough money. If I have to pay emotionally, he should at least pay financially," said Pam. "I must admit I like having this power over him. Now he can get a taste of his own medicine. I'm still not sure whether I'll tell on him. But I got the most expensive therapist I could and I see her twice a week!"

The others laughed. "Great idea," Terry commented. "Hell, why should they get off the hook?"

"For me, all this spills over into my present life too," Denise observed. "The feelings of panic and fear that I have almost constantly are familiar. I vividly remember feeling this way all through my childhood. I mean, the incest was a problem but it happened in an already screwed-up house. So now it brings up all those issues too and I can see how they play out in my relationships with men I date and with my kids."

"I still can't get over the betrayal," added Linda. "I had always adored my uncle. I didn't get much attention from my parents, they were busy with my older sister who was always getting into trouble. Pete was the one who gave me any affection and attention. He lived in a nearby city so I saw him pretty often.

"I can't remember an exact first time but we were always very affectionate with each other, very huggy and I always snuggled with him. I would spend the night at his house sometimes. His wife wasn't around much but she was always pretty nice to me. But one time when I stayed over at his house, after I went to bed, I heard my bedroom door open. I pretended to be asleep. I could tell it was him from the footsteps. He climbed into bed with me and started fondling me. I didn't know what was going on but it didn't seem right so I just kept pretending to be asleep. Then he got up and left the room and I just laid there the rest of the night, wide awake, trying to figure out what had just happened.

"The next morning he acted like he always had but I found myself staying away from him. Then at one point we were watching TV together and he told me to snuggle up. I said I didn't want to but he moved over to me and pulled me to him. He put his arm around me and then started gently rubbing my breasts. I had just started developing so I was really embarrassed and tried to pull away. He was very calm and quiet and said that since I was developing, I needed to learn what to do when I went on dates. I said I was never going to date so I didn't need to learn anything. I really felt nervous. I got up and said I needed to get something. Before I left the room he said, 'This is something just between us, sweetheart. It's only OK to do it if we always keep it our secret. And don't ever tell your mother. If you do, she'll be very jealous and it would kill her.' I left the room and didn't return. After that, I didn't stay over at his house anymore and I tried to steer clear of him whenever he came to visit. I didn't exactly know how I felt about him after that but I knew I could never tell anyone and even if I did, they probably wouldn't believe me. But I could never trust him again and I never wanted to be around him after that."

"You know," said Meredith, "it's that loss of trust that has really screwed up my life. For me, it was my brother who abused me. He's 4 years older than me. It started when he was about 13 and he said he had a big date coming up and he wanted to practice what to do with the girl. So he asked me if I'd help him. I didn't know what he was talking about but we always got along, so I said sure. So we go in his room and he tells me to sit on his bed, and he tries to kiss me, I mean with his tongue. I was grossed out and told him to stop. But he said he really needed my help and if I did it, he'd buy me a record I had wanted. But he made me swear I would never tell anyone about it, that no one would understand, especially our parents. So I knew it must be wrong. But I really wanted that record so I stayed. Anyway, we kissed and he fondled me some. That was about it. And then we went to the record store and he bought me the record. A few weeks later, he wanted to do it again but I said no. Then he threatened to tell on me. I reminded him about why he had told me not to tell but he said our folks would believe him because it was OK for boys to fool around but only girls who were sluts did, especially with their own brother. I wasn't sure about this logic but I was only about 9. And I didn't know what a slut was but from the way he said it, I was sure I didn't want to be one. And I knew it would be humiliating if he told. So we did it again. He didn't bother me again for about a month and then he wanted to do it. But this time, I'm not sure why, I said if he made me do it again, I'd tell and then he'd be in trouble. He wasn't sure if I was lying but I guess he decided it wasn't worth risking because he didn't try to do it again after that. He also had a girlfriend by then and I think they were messing around so he didn't need me anymore. And that kind of upset me because then I felt used and like he didn't care about me anymore. Talk about screwed up! I still can't trust people and I'm still mad as hell about it."

DeAnne nodded. "The anger is a big thing for me. It's ruined most of my relationships with friends and lovers. I feel like I have this huge rage inside me, that if it ever got out, it would be homicidal. I think it's really anger and rage toward what happened, toward my father for doing it and my mother for not protecting me. But I tend to turn it inward and then I get extremely depressed. And I know I have a wall up and people can't get close to me. I hate that but I don't feel like I can risk getting close to anyone. It's too scary. I couldn't stand being betrayed again so I just go along until someone starts to get close and then I break it off. I've had trouble at work too. My boss has told me several times that I have an attitude problem and I'm real irritable with my coworkers. She's right but I can't seem to control it. Sometimes I feel like there's so much rage, I'm going to explode." They all nodded in agreement.

"I know what you mean," said Jenny, "and it screws up every relationship I've ever been in. I've been married once, lived with guys twice, I always seem to end up with guys who beat me around. I hate it but I feel like I deserve it. I've got two kids, a girl 16 and a boy 14. They're wild. They've never had a stable home life. They've had a lot of my anger dumped on them. I'm ashamed to say it but when they were younger, I knocked them around a bit. I mean, I never really hurt them but they must have been scared to death. They pretty much come and go as they please now and they don't listen to me at all. I know my daughter's messing around because I found birth control pills in her room. I was snooping, I know I shouldn't have been, because I thought she might be on drugs. I didn't find drugs but I found the pills. I confronted her and we had a big fight and it came out that she's been sleeping around since she was 14. And it turns out that my son, at 14, has tried some drugs. What a mess. I can't blame it all on my incest but I'm sure it made a mess even messier."

"Have you tried counseling with the kids?" asked Rachel.

"Yeah," Jenny responded. "I've tried to get them to go but they refuse to. They both say I'm the one with the problem and to leave them alone." She was crying hard as she reached for the box of Kleenex.

"It's really horrible," Terry agreed. "My kids are grown and gone now but I don't hear from them much. They don't sound too different from yours, Jenny. I was with their dad for about 10 years. It started out OK, although I was pregnant when we got married. But after a couple of years he started having affairs and I got involved with a woman at work. I had never had a lesbian affair before that but it just happened and, in so many ways, it was just a lot easier and more comfortable. My husband found out about it, took the kids, and filed for divorce. Patty and I stayed together for about 6 years. She had been physically and sexually abused when she was a kid so we had some things in common. But we were both so needy, we just couldn't make it work. I haven't been with anyone since then. I just can't handle close relationships."

"Until I went to college, I think I was basically asexual. In high school, I ran with the fast crowd. I drank a lot and smoked grass and hash and did acid but sex never entered my thoughts," remarked Marsha. "Then, my first year at college, I realized I wasn't attracted to men. I don't think it had anything to do with being abused. They just didn't do anything for me. I ended up getting involved with a woman who lived in my dorm. It didn't last long but I knew then that I was a lesbian."

Over in a corner, Carla was quietly crying. The others turned to her and she spoke. "My husband's a good guy. I lived with another guy for a long time until I met Steve. I fell for him hard. He works hard and he's been really supportive while I've been going through all of this. We have two boys, 9 and 6, and a 4-year-old girl. And they all love me, but sometimes I feel like I hate them, really hate them. And it's just because they're males. It feels like there's a pretty big part of me that hates all men because of what happened to me. I know I shouldn't, but I do. It scares me because when I feel that angry, I get worried that I might take it out on them, like hit the kids or something. And I know I'm nicer and more patient with Cheryl and it's not because she's a girl but because she's *not* a boy. Does that make any sense?"

"Does it ever," said Gina. "I had never thought about it like that before but that's exactly how I feel. I'm sure that's a major reason for my divorce and why I stay away from getting in a committed relationship. I like the sex and I like the companionship but only on my terms. Maybe it has to do with control. I have to control the relationship completely or I can't stand it. Maybe since I had no control over my stepfather, I somehow decided I'd never allow myself to be out of control with a man again. And I did fine with my kids when they were little and they'd do exactly what I wanted them to do. As long as I could control them. But once they started having minds of their own, we started having huge fights. They're grown today and we don't talk to each other much. This is amazing. This is the first time I've ever made this connection."

"Boy, just thinking about how it's affected all of us and our relationships as adults makes me furious," said Mary. "I'm so full of rage, I just don't know what to do with it."

"I like to take a pillow and slam it into the sofa as hard as I can," offered Julie. "I name it Bill, after him, and yell and scream. I just hope the neighbors never hear me!"

"We live about an hour and a half from a huge amusement park," said Linda. "When it's open in the summer, I go and ride all the big roller coasters. I can scream as loud as I want and I fit right in. I do it all day long and by the end of the day, my throat is hoarse but I feel better. I just wish they were open during the winter."

"That's a great idea. I love roller coasters. My problem is that I don't do anything about my anger so it just builds and builds and then I end up yelling at my husband and my kids and the dog. These are some great ideas," Meredith said.

Carol spoke up. "Hitting the sofa helps me too but I think my therapy has made the biggest difference. It's really tough to relive what happened but it seems to help me put my anger where it belongs. I definitely feel less rage since I've been seeing my therapist."

"But I don't have enough money for private therapy," said Peggy. "I don't have a job, all I get is welfare. I live in a one-bedroom apartment with my 6-year-old son. My ex hardly ever sends me any money. Paying somebody $80 an hour or more every week is out of the question. But I like the pillow idea."

"Peggy," offered Leigh, "there's counseling available on a sliding scale and the Rape Crisis Center runs support groups for free. There are lots of resources available that don't cost anything that you could use. I'll get you a list and phone numbers." Several other women asked Leigh to make extra copies for all of them.

For a while, it was quiet. Some of the women were crying, some were hugging, some were squeezing each other's hands, some were fidgeting. It had been an intense and moving morning for all of them. They knew they were not alone and that they were not crazy. "These are incredibly strong and brave women," Rachel thought to herself. "I admire their courage and their unwillingness to remain victims. I feel cautiously hopeful for each of them."

CONCLUSION

The impact of incest does not end once the abusive act does. Its aftereffects permeate the survivor's life and can affect, for example, her self-concept, her ability to trust and form successful adult relationships, and her coping skills. The defenses that allowed her to cope with the trauma as a child can continue into adulthood, where they are no longer appropriate or functional. As a child, the messages she received from her perpetrator were designed to coerce her into keeping the secret and blaming herself. As an adult, messages from significant others may invalidate her reality and challenge the veracity of her experiences or they may be validating and supportive.

Support from other survivors is often extremely helpful, as they find that they are not alone, that their emotional upheaval is related to the abuse, and that they can recover. What began with each woman's courage to break the conspiracy of silence (Butler, 1978) has become a louder voice as survivors find each other and share their stories. Through their willingness to speak out, individually and collectively, they confront and challenge the stigma of their past and shape the future for all of our children.

RELEVANT CONCEPTS

betrayal of trust
conspiracy of silence
incest

long-term impact
personal control
relational concerns
social support

DISCUSSION QUESTIONS

1. What themes were evident as the women shared their stories. Were any differences apparent? If so, what were they and how did they impact the survivors?

2. What are the risks for a survivor confronting her perpetrator? Telling her family of her abuse? Telling close friends? Acquaintances?

3. Why might other survivors be perceived as more supportive than close friends who were not survivors? When might support from nonsurvivors be important?

4. What are some ways for survivors to deal with their rage?

5. If a close friend or relative had been sexually abused by a relative, and you were the first person she told, what would you do?

REFERENCES/SUGGESTED READINGS

Bass, E., & Davis, L. (1994). *The courage to heal: A guide for women survivors of child sexual abuse* (3rd ed.). New York: Harper & Row.

Butler, S. (1978). *The conspiracy of silence: The trauma of incest.* San Francisco: New Glide Publications.

Courtois, C. A. (1988). *Healing the incest wound: Adult survivors in therapy.* New York: Norton.

Crewdson, J. (1988). *By silence betrayed.* Boston: Little, Brown.

Dinsmore, C. (1991). *From surviving to thriving: Incest, feminism, and recovery.* Albany: State University of New York Press.

Poston, C., & Lison, K. (1989). *Reclaiming our lives: Hope for adult survivors of incest.* Boston: Little, Brown.

Ray, E. B. (1996). Challenging the stigmatizing messages: The emerging voices of adult survivors of incest. In E. B. Ray (Ed.), *Communication and disenfranchisement: Social health issues and implications* (pp. 273–291). Mahwah, NJ: Lawrence Erlbaum Associates.

Russell, D. E. H. (1986). *The secret trauma: Incest in the lives of girls and women.* New York: Basic Books.

11 *To Love, Honor, and Obey: One Woman's Narrative of Intimate Violence*

Lisa Kanae
University of Hawaii

James T. West
Honolulu, Hawaii

It was a typical Tuesday morning at the hospital. I started recording minutes for the weekly staff meeting. I was 26 years old and had worked as the department's secretary for 4 years. My boss smiled at me from across the conference room table. She always thanked me for being stable, competent, and efficient. She trusted me.

About a half hour into the meeting I started to feel lightheaded and nauseous. My vision grew distorted then gradually faded away. The only sounds I heard were snatches of comments coming from a colorless haze hovering above my face.

"She looked fine this morning. . . ."

"I know she's had some personal problems. . . ."

"You think it's drugs? . . ."

"She never talks about it. . . ."

"Get her to the ER!"

Someone lifted me into a wheelchair. The emergency room was only one floor down from the conference room. I had tried to pretend this was just another Tuesday morning.

The Beginning of the End

I remained silent as they wheeled me down the hospital corridor. Puzzled coworkers searched my face for answers, but I no longer had the strength to make up excuses and I was in too much pain to feel embarrassed. The only person I wanted was my husband, but that was impossible because he couldn't be trusted. Besides, I had to protect him. I thought of how embarrassed he would be if I dared to say anything to anyone. I had to protect the secrets I kept hidden beneath the bruises on my body. Now, however, the lies I had accumulated over the years could no longer be hidden.

The ER staff started yelling at me. "Are you pregnant?" "Do you have a history of substance abuse?" "Are you taking any kind of medication? . . ." "Her blood pressure is up there—170 over 100. Set up an EKG monitor."

I prayed to myself, please, let me keep my blouse on. With the impulse of a knee-jerk reflex, I instantly made up a story as the nurse lifted my blouse up over my head. I wanted to be able to explain where the bruises came from.

No one knew about the Valium and Prozac I took to veil my anguish. I blamed job stress or PMS for my anxiety so I could get medication without a hint of impropriety. The day before I had received compliments on my weight loss and pretended to be proud. The truth was I stopped eating 3 weeks ago so my husband would have less and less of me to hate. It was as if I believed that one day he would have nothing left to shove, hit, and humiliate. I thought maybe then he could love me. I started to grow faint again.

Fifteen minutes passed. I was cold, hooked up to an EKG monitor, and naked from the waist up. The bruises on my upper body and arms were exposed. I felt as if the entire hospital had discovered the shame and embarrassment I successfully hid and denied for years. A nurse stood next to my bed. Her smile was genuine and sympathetic. I realized that I could not pretend I fell down or tripped over something; I could not pretend I didn't hurt, and I could not pretend it would never happen again.

The Turning Point

I heard a wheezing sound behind the partition next to me. There was an old woman lying on her back with her mouth wide open. Her complexion was sallow, her hair a brittle gray. She looked like she was dying. I wondered if she wanted to live. An overwhelming compassion for this woman replaced whatever anguish I felt. I felt her powerlessness and wanted to give her the strength to fight back. But she couldn't feel my empathy. She couldn't feel anything anymore.

I asked myself at what point in my marriage did I decide to stop feeling. At what point did I give up on myself? This woman behind the partition was old, very sick, with no one to help her. I was young, relatively healthy, with no one to help me. Yet, I had the capability to stand up and walk away. How many violent fights and humiliating remarks will it take to make me as numb as she is? I realized I needed to choose between confronting the pain of my abusive marriage or denying the death of my spirit.

I sat up, got dressed, walked up to the nurses' station, and insisted on leaving. No one was waiting for me and I had no one to call. Years of isolation left me far removed from family and friends. I refused to call my husband. I left the hospital wondering who the old woman was, wondering how I could make up for the years I wasted dying in an abusive marriage; and I wondered where I was going to go.

For the first time in many years I felt free. I walked toward the nearest bus stop. A bus approached, but I was afraid it wasn't the right one. I instinctively started to hesitate, but then I remembered the strained wheezing sound of the old woman's breathing. I pictured the pale color of her skin. I felt her helplessness. I told myself any bus will start me off in the right direction; just get on one. I climbed into the bus, found my place among the crowd, and began my journey.

Why do women stay in abusive relationships? Ever since I started college and married my husband I had tried to rationalize and justify my husband's behavior, all the while believing that he cared about my welfare and safety. Quite a paradoxical statement, but it exemplifies the stark contradictions one confronts in the face of an abusive person who happens to be the man you love—who happens to be your husband. The typical cycle of abuse and sweetness fused a formidable bond between my husband and me. Years of conditioning turned our relationship into a complex snarl that distorted the difference between tenderness and cruelty. As the years passed the physical and emotional abuse became the norm for both of us.

When I left the emergency room I realized that all of the anger, confusion, and love, yes, love as I knew it, was no longer worth protecting. For the first time in many years I truly owned my thoughts and decisions. This wasn't easy for me. Although my husband wasn't physically present, his pervasive control made the simple decision to get on a bus a difficult and frightening one. But I got on the bus and the journey to find myself has been the most challenging and rewarding experience of my adult life.

Recalling the Relationship

I hardly knew who I was before that day in the emergency room. At one time I believed the wedding vows I took before God and family made up the core of my identity. My secret battle began the day I vowed to love, honor, and obey my husband. I was 21 years old and too inexperienced and immature to understand the profound depth of those vows. I simply repeated the words love, honor, and obey as spontaneously as you would begin a fairy tale with "once upon a time." Like the romantic love stories I read when I was a little girl, those vows gave me hope. The handsome prince chose me over all the other eligible young maidens, which meant I was very special. The fact that someone loved me gave me a reason to exist.

Ironically enough, our courtship was the result of a car accident that took place one morning during rush hour traffic. I smashed the front end of my Volkswagen into a car in front of me. My exhusband was the patrolman who calmed my nerves and took control of the chaos. He rescued the young, helpless maiden. He was 28 years old, confident, clean-cut, athletic, and articulate—a far cry from the boys I dated who were typically my own age. He knew how to make me feel beautiful, cherished, and safe. Within a few weeks our attraction for one another grew so intense we immediately mistook it for love.

Within a month Doug left for Micronesia. He planned to start a security company there and was determined to continue our courtship through letters and phone calls. I received a letter every day for 3 months. My entire understanding of this man was conceptualized through his letters to me. I saw in him everything a young woman could want in a man. He was romantic, devoted, sensitive, ambitious, and solid. Within 6 months, I agreed to move to Micronesia and marry someone I thought I knew. It was a wild, romantic venture I could not resist. The relative amount of risk did not frighten me at all. Not only did I have a passion for adventure, I was also cursed with naive idealism. I simply believed that, together, my husband and I would conquer the world and live happily ever after.

My parents divorced when I was 9 years old. My mother, being a single parent, struggled to support my brother and me by holding down two jobs. She worked very hard waiting on tables and was never home. I grew up wanting to be part of a "real" family, one that stayed together. I vowed never to become another divorce statistic the way my parents did. I was certain that I could create a real family with Doug, my handsome prince.

He was a born-again Christian and felt it was necessary that I, too, be born again. I was impressed by this young man's religious convictions and his belief in God. I envisioned the perfect marriage held together by the glue of traditional Christian values. How could anything go wrong if your spouse was a good Christian man? I figured I was safe at last.

We had our first big argument about 3 days after the wedding during a party at his friend's house. There were a few single men there, one of whom I had a passing conversation with. Doug saw me laughing with this man and immediately grabbed my arm, pulled me into a room, and slammed the door shut.

He gripped my shoulders and shook me the way an enraged parent shakes an unruly child. He was so angry he could hardly speak without punching a wall or clutching a pillow. He blatantly accused me of flirting with the young man outside. I embarrassed him because my conduct was not that of a good wife, but a whore.

A whore? I was more stunned by that word than I was frightened by my husband's temper. I argued with him and tried to defend myself, but not only was this useless, it exacerbated his temper. He simply refused to listen to me. The fact is I belonged to him and I could not go on teasing other men with a smile or witty conversation. Most of all, I should remember that my behavior was a reflection of the man I married. Solid men do not want to marry flirtatious or promiscuous women.

How could I do such a thing to him in front of his friends? How could I not realize how much I hurt him? Why didn't I know better than to disappoint or embarrass him this way? This incident was the first of many in which I embarrassed and displeased my husband.

As the months went by, other small, innocent actions were described as wrong and bad. The fact that I didn't know I was doing anything wrong left me paralyzed. I became so paranoid that every step I took was like walking onto a wobbly old bridge. I never knew what to expect.

Who was this man yelling at me so often with so much intensity? He certainly wasn't the handsome, gentle prince whom I thought I had married. He was a stern brutal officer enforcing his law. But each time after he verbally punished me he would apologize. He loved me so much, he said. He would look defeated and I would feel guilty. We would hold each other and say that we would work things out.

Our fights had dramatic highs followed by gratifying lows. The intense tenderness that always followed the extreme anger was like a drug. We eventually grew dependent on these emotional roller coaster rides, which strengthened the bond between us. These fights left me exhausted and I eventually agreed to try my best to change. After all, I loved him and all I really wanted was for him to love me. Once I resigned to his wishes, he always rewarded me with affection and sex. If I refused to submit, he would not speak to me or touch me for days at a time.

Our first years together shattered my dreams of what marriage should be. Doug assumed this paternal role that I found difficult to tolerate. Everything I did was monitored and corrected if need be, from the clothes I wore to the kind of music I listened to. I constantly challenged his authority, sometimes just in spite. I was a spunky, strong-willed young woman with more energy than he expected. I realize now that I slipped into the role of rebellious child, which impulsively encouraged his assumed role as parent.

I accused him of trying to change me from a spirited, attractive young woman to a matronly wallflower. He said I was being impossible and too stupid to see the obvious solution to our problems. If I did what I was told and stopped resisting then he wouldn't get angry. Of course the justification for his control was love. He was responsible for my welfare and safety. He just wanted what was best for me. The truth is, if I followed suit I would be less of a burden upon his deep insecurities.

He mentioned once that he wished I was more like his mother. She never questioned his father's opinions or decisions and she always did what she was told. Because she was such a good woman his father treated her like a queen. Doug often suggested other role models I should aspire to. There were a few women who attended the church we went to whom I should socialize with and learn from.

They were passive women who never got involved with community or church programs and never attracted much attention. Whenever Doug and I fought about my inappropriate behavior, he always hurled these women's names at me. Why can't you be more like Catherine or Karen, he'd say; they never contradict their husband's opinions in public or refuse to do what they are told.

No matter how hard I tried to fit the mold, bits and pieces of the real me always seemed to spill out at the wrong time. During a dinner conversation with another couple, I contradicted Doug's opinion about homosexuality, which he abhorred. It wasn't a direct attack on Doug's opinion, I simply said I had several gay friends. Nevertheless, I was contradicting his values in front of other people. He called me an idiot. I simply wasn't knowledgeable enough about the subject to have my own opinion. As far as he was concerned, I wasn't smart enough to have an opinion about anything. He laughed to buffer the uncomfortable mood he created at the dinner table. This humiliated me even more.

The minute we got into the car he started yelling at me. Naturally I argued back—I was entitled to my own opinion. When I told him he was being unreasonable he grabbed the hair on the back of my head and pushed my face into the dashboard. He called me a rebellious punk who didn't know shit about the world. I was too frightened to cry or fight back and remained silent until we got home. My silence never aggravated him.

That night I went to bed alone while Doug read. He sat in his favorite chair in the living room. The only light in the house came from the reading lamp on the table next to him. I lay in bed and searched the dark for answers. We were up all night. At sunrise he walked into the bedroom, sat down beside me, and started to cry. He was sorry and promised to never hurt me again. His embrace seemed so genuine—so tortured with guilt. I finally broke down and wept. Like refugees afraid to face the future, we spent the entire morning hidden in that bedroom.

Through the years he repeatedly broke his promise, only to whisper it to me over and over again. His business took off and he spent most of his time at the office. I found a job managing a dental office, established a close circle of friends, and spent most of my time at work. We eventually grew in different directions, which finally provided a little bit of peace and happiness at home.

However, his need to control our relationship repeatedly led to more intimate violence. One day he told me that I couldn't even make a tuna-melt sandwich right. When I put the plate down in front of him, he went into a rage. I didn't toast the bread right, he said. He called me an incompetent idiot and threw the entire sandwich at me. He stomped out of the house, slammed the door behind him and left the melted cheese clinging to the kitchen cabinets for me to clean up.

The periods of peace between these fights were so sweet I often buried the hurt and enjoyed the happiness as best I could. When we found the time to do things together we did the things most young couples did. We owned a small Hobie catamaran and enjoyed sailing the isolated waters along the south coast of the island. We hiked, snorkeled, and frequented a tacky little Chinese restaurant.

Doug and I put up such a convincing front that I was certain no one imagined what was happening in our home. He seemed so charming and gentle in the company of others, whereas I grew more introverted and meek. Whenever I found the courage to question his abusive behavior, he blamed me for being so unhappy and unsatisfied. I was too sensitive and blew every little thing out of proportion. He said I constantly made him feel inadequate. It never occurred to me that Doug felt so awful about himself. He seemed to have everything in control, including me.

By our 5th-year anniversary, Doug's personality darkened. He complained about how frustrating it was to do business within the islands' corrupt political environment. He could not deal with the stress and eventually took it out on me. His mood swings got worse and so did the violence. He started shoving me against walls, pushing me down on the ground, pulling my hair, and occasionally kicking me. Sometimes I hit back and felt awful inside. I didn't realize I had it in me to actually strike another person. Sometimes I did nothing and just took whatever he dished out. I hid the bruises well. He never hit my face. Friends sensed his dark, pensive moods but I denied everything. I was so ashamed.

I secretly kept a journal, mainly for self-therapy. One of my entries revealed my desire to leave. When Doug found the journal he was furious. It hurt him to read about my anguish, my wanting to escape. He tore up the pages, threw them in my face, and said I didn't have the courage to follow through. He was right—I was petrified. He threatened to kill me if I tried to run away. I believed him and he sensed my fear. He took me into his arms, begged me to stay, and sobbed. If he lost me, he would have nothing to live for. I was his life. The handsome prince turned into a helpless child. I held him for a long time, stroked his hair, and promised to never leave him.

But if I had never left him, I would probably not be alive today. I woke up in the emergency room. I realized that his need to control me with verbal and physical abuse would never change.

OTHER WOMEN'S NARRATIVES OF INTIMATE VIOLENCE

Although every woman's experience with intimate violence is unique, my (first author) story illustrates some of the common threads that are found in most violent relationships. As in my case, intimate violence is always preceded by a long period of verbal abuse. The verbal abuse breaks down the woman's self-esteem and makes her try harder to make the relationship work. Whereas the man tries different strategies to force the woman to relinquish control of the relationship, the woman tries to understand his anger and keep the marriage together.

America's cultural and media traditions position the family as a sacred institution. These traditions are reinforced in rhetorical practices on numerous levels within our society, and are especially clear in the way women's narratives position the institution of family as so important that even numerous violent incidents are not enough to force them to leave their relationships. Women describe leaving a relationship as literally an unthinkable act. Their self-image is fused to an image of marriage and family.

Research on the narratives of women who experience intimate violence also shows how women experience great ideological pressures from church authorities, counselors, and family members who advise them to remain in their violent marriages (West, 1995). In addition to the institutional voices, the violence in the relationship is also used as a means to keep individuals from leaving the relationship. When a husband tells his wife he will kill her if she tries to leave, she takes those threats seriously because he has repeatedly shown her that he has no qualms about using violence.

Nowhere was the use of violence to control a relationship more publicly evident than in the Nicole Simpson case. On June 22, 1995, as O.J. Simpson sat in a jail cell awaiting pretrial proceedings, the L.A. police released a 911 tape of an intimate violence incident between O.J. and Nicole that took place on October 25, 1993. In the telephone call to the 911 dispatcher, we heard Nicole reporting that O.J. had broken down her back door. We also heard O.J. threatening to beat her, a threat she took very seriously because he had beaten her on at least nine occasions throughout their marriage. As O.J. is threatening to kill her in the background, we hear the police dispatcher ask Nicole what she had done wrong that O.J. would want to harm her. This 15-minute tape was played on every local and national TV and radio news program repeatedly for several days and nights.

One of the positive side-effects of this intense media exposure was that shelters and hot lines for abused women reported a huge increase in the number of calls they received from women who became willing for the first time to discuss the violence in their relationships. Intimate violence became the number one topic in the mass media throughout the United States for several weeks because of this highly dramatic case.

I could have easily ended up being killed by my husband. But I did nothing wrong. I didn't deserve to be beaten. No woman or man or child deserves to be beaten, no matter what they did. Violence is always an excuse to try to gain control of other people. It is the ultimate form of control.

As my husband took more control of our relationship, first through verbal abuse and then through physical force, I came to think of the violence as my fault. I thought that I had actually done something wrong and deserved to be beaten. Only coming face to face with my own death forced me to leave the relationship.

Except for my violent relationship, I think of myself as normal in every way. Unfortunately, violent relationships seem to be almost a "normal" experience for many women in America. Each day throughout the United States, police departments file hundreds of reports of husbands killing, maiming, and beating their wives. In Los Angeles in 1993, there were 20,000 cases of intimate violence. Each year, thousands of these cases throughout the United States result in someone being murdered. We must stop asking why women stay in violent relationships or why some men use violence against women. Instead, we need to ask why men are violent and why women are so easily victimized. And we need to recognize the irony that, after being so thoroughly socialized to think of their place as the home, it is the victims, rather than the abusers, who are expected to leave (Hoff, 1990). To help women break the cycle of violence, they must be given support, individually, collectively, and culturally, that shows them that no sacred vows or institutional or cultural practices require them to tolerate violence.

RELEVANT CONCEPTS

cultural practices
cycle of violence
emotional abuse
ideology of violence
intimate violence
relational control
sacred vows

DISCUSSION QUESTIONS

1. What was the relationship process that Lisa describes as leading to the violence? Were there indications during the courtship that she was entering an abusive relationship?

2. What actions or support systems may help prevent or stop the cycle of intimate violence?

3. How do people in violent relationships smooth over the contradictions between being in "love" and also being verbally and physically abused?

4. What cultural practices make intimate violence such a common experience in America?

REFERENCES/SUGGESTED READINGS

Foucault, M. (1980). *Power/knowledge* (C. Gordon, Ed.). New York: Pantheon.

Gelles, R., & Straus, M. (1989). *Intimate violence*. New York: Simon & Schuster.

Gordon, L. (1988). *Heroes of their own lives*. New York: Viking.

Hoff, L. A. (1990). *Battered women as survivors*. London: Routledge.

Walker, L. (1984). *The battered woman syndrome*. New York: Springer.

West, J. (1995). Understanding how the dynamics of ideology influence violence between intimates. In S. Duck & J. Wood (Eds.), *Confronting relationship challenges* (pp. 129–149). Thousand Oaks, CA: Sage.

12 *Sexual Harassment: Raising Consciousness and Sharing Solutions*

Timothy J. Hack
Lafayette, Indiana

Robin P. Clair
Purdue University

Nicole reviewed the details in her mind as she rode the elevator up to Mr. Powers' office. Mr. Powers was the president of the Boston office of the architectural firm, Hale and Hale. It was an unscheduled meeting.

He had phoned her at her desk and inquired if she had the time to go over the plans of the Kompten Building project. Of course she did. When the boss of your boss calls about a project, you make the time, especially when it is your first "real job" since graduating from college.

Mr. Powers' secretary was not at her desk. This didn't surprise Nicole. It was 12:15 p.m. and most everybody was at lunch. Nicole herself had been halfway out the door to catch a chicken salad at the small "gulp and choke" they called a deli in the lobby of the office building.

As Nicole entered the conference room, she was a little surprised that no one else was there. She took this as a sign that her work was acceptable. If there were any problems with her design, she figured her supervisor would be sitting in on this meeting.

Nicole was eager to do the best job possible. Her work, prior to this project, was done in conjunction with other architects. This was the first time she was given responsibility for a complete job from start to finish. Granted, it was only a two-story parking garage and not the Ritz Hotel, but it was all hers to design.

Nicole spread the blueprints out on the highly polished oak table in the middle of the room. She mentally computed the square feet of the table. The figure she arrived at was nearly the same as her working cubicle.

Mr. Powers entered from the door leading to his office.

"Nicole, I'm glad you were able to come up on such short notice. I hope this didn't interrupt any lunch plans?" questioned Mr. Powers, as he reached for Nicole's hand. Rather than extending a firm handshake, Mr. Powers held Nicole's hand between both of his hands. They stood like that for a moment.

"No. I . . . I already had a bite to eat at my desk," fibbed Nicole, a little flustered by her boss holding her hand. She didn't want to be impolite and pull her hand away, even though she was uncomfortable.

"Good, let's take a look at these plans." He directed her to the first chair from the head of the table. He pulled the chair out for her and then lightly placed his hands on her shoulders. Glancing up, Nicole wasn't sure if Mr. Powers was looking at the blueprints on the table or down the front of her blouse. Nicole felt her muscles tighten as he kept his hands on her shoulders.

With Mr. Powers standing directly behind and above her, Nicole began to feel self-conscious about the blouse she had chosen to wear. It had a scalloped neck, which was fine when she was sitting straight in her chair or standing. However, she would need to lean over to point out particular features in the blueprints. The loose overlap of the blouse would gap slightly. Nothing very risqué, but more skin would be revealed than Nicole normally intended.

Nicole remembered a class she had in her final year in college. It was during the year of the Clarence Thomas hearings. She remembered the heated discussion that had erupted in class when a student mockingly remarked on Anita Hill's accusations. Suddenly, everyone had an opinion or a story to tell. Nicole heard the story about the woman who accused a male coworker of sexual harassment, only to be reprimanded herself by the management for wearing suggestive clothing to work. The managers believed that she created the environment that encouraged the harassment.

Nicole remembered the reaction from the woman sitting next to her in class, who always wore low-cut tank tops. She adamantly claimed that she could wear what she "blank" well wanted to and that didn't give any man the right to harass her.

Another student claimed that in the workplace women shouldn't show any more skin than a man does in a business suit. This prompted a student to point out that some companies maintain a policy that a woman must wear a knee-length dress to the office.

Nicole didn't care what she had to wear. Her dream was to be an architect and if that meant wearing a sack cloth to work she would do it. The discussion did make her aware that what she wore might reflect on her competence as an architect.

It was Helen, the director of benefits at Hale and Hale, who helped Nicole by becoming her mentor. She suggested to Nicole that if she didn't want to risk any kind of negative response she should wear "Murphy Brown clothes" to work. That meant high neckline, long sleeves, dresses to the knee.

This morning it happened that the white blouse she normally wore with this outfit was at the cleaners. In a rush she substituted this one. She hadn't any client meetings scheduled for today. So she didn't give it another thought, at least not until Mr. Powers had stood over her.

After Mr. Powers gave her shoulders a little squeeze, he sat at the head of the table.

Nicole began to explain the details of the plan to Mr. Powers. She pointed out the changes she had made, due to a supplier having an inadequate inventory of a particular item. Mr. Powers questioned the wisdom of this decision and asked if she had explored alternative options.

Nicole quickly defended her decision. Leaning over she pointed to the affected area in the blueprints. In the middle of her argument she looked up to see her boss looking down her blouse.

"You have some very good points there," said Mr. Powers with a slow smile.

Nicole immediately straightened up. Her cheeks began to turn red. She felt like somebody had turned the temperature up 10° in the conference room.

"That's why I made the decision to make that substitution," Nicole finished abruptly.

Mr. Powers leaned forward, looked down at the blueprints, and then back up at Nicole. His eyes lingered for a brief second at her chest. Looking her in the eyes he said, "I like the work you're doing. If you continue to make the right decisions," here his eyes glanced at her chest again, "you will do very well in this company. I think you should keep me abreast of this project." He smiled. "Plan on meeting with me here every week at this time to go over the details. You don't want to disappoint," he paused again, "Mr. Kompten."

Mr. Powers slid his chair back, stood up, towered over Nicole for a second, and then departed through the door to his office.

Nicole sat there stunned. Her mind swirled with random thoughts and conflicting emotions. In a daze, she rolled up the blueprints. The trip back to her desk seemed like a series of snapshots.

* * *

Snapshot - She is standing in front of the elevator.

Snapshot - She is in the elevator, the door opens, people get out; she never saw them get on.

Snapshot - She is sitting at her desk.

Snapshot - She is in the ladies' room, pacing.

That is where Helen found her.

"Nicole, what's the matter?" Helen gently inquired. Helen sat on the couch. She motioned for Nicole to stop her pacing, and to sit next to her.

Nicole sat and took a deep breath.

"I'll try to explain," she began. "I'm not sure what happened. I mean I know what happened, but I'm not sure I can put it into words."

"Just try," Helen encouraged her.

"It started out as a normal meeting with Mr. Powers," Nicole said, looking at the floor. "I was pretty excited to have a meeting with him about my Kompten project. You know the one I've been working so hard on. But, somehow things changed. I mean he took my hand, but he didn't actually shake it. He just held it between his two hands for the longest time. And I just about crawled out of my skin when he put his hands on my shoulders. Later he stared at my chest. It was only for a second, but that second seemed like an eternity. And he said some things that . . . ," Nicole's voice trailed off.

Nicole started talking again, her voice flat. "He wants me to meet with him once a week." She paused and looked at Helen. "I don't think I could be in a crowded room with him."

Nicole suddenly questioned Helen. "My work. What about my project? Did I get that project because I deserved it, or did he give it to me so he could get me alone with him?"

"Don't undermine your abilities. You are an excellent architect," asserted Helen.

"I never should have worn this blouse," muttered Nicole.

"Don't be silly," countered Helen.

"But if I hadn't worn this blouse, he wouldn't have had the opportunity to look down my blouse. It's my fault."

"Absolutely not! Didn't you say he started the meeting by holding your hand a little too long, and didn't he place his hands on your shoulders?"

"Yes."

"Then remember," Helen continued forcefully. "You didn't do anything wrong. You are the victim of his lecherousness."

Helen stood up. "Now, why don't you go home. Write down everything that happened. Tomorrow is Saturday. I'm having lunch with a friend I think you should meet. Can you join us tomorrow?"

Nicole agreed that she didn't think she could keep her mind on her work. She thought lunch tomorrow would be fine.

* * *

When she returned to her desk, Helen called Carol Thomas, an old friend and former coworker. She wasn't able to get through to her so she left a message with Carol's secretary to call her back at the office before five o'clock or at home after seven.

After she hung up the phone, Helen pondered Nicole's dilemma. She was sure that at this point in time even Nicole did not realize that she was at a crossroads and would have some very difficult decisions to make. Decisions she probably never imagined she would have to make in her whole life. Through no fault of her own, Nicole's life and career were about to change.

Helen deplored the situation that Mr. Powers had created. She felt that sexual harassment, whether obvious or subtle, is insidious.

Helen was reminded of incidents that happened to her when she first started to work. A lot of the blatant harassment was now gone, but obviously not all. She could remember calendars with near-naked women on them, hanging in every office from the president of the company to the mail clerk. Some of the men, at that time, participated in the sexual humiliation of women as an office sport.

Helen decided, early in her career, to confront the abuse and harassment in her own way. She felt she had a good sense of humor and a quick wit. She employed these methods when confronted with sexual harassment.

Helen remembered the time when she had just started with the company as a secretary. She arrived at work one day, to find the men in the office moving all the desks and file cabinets. They told her they wanted to arrange the office in a more efficient manner. Her desk ended up in front of the blower for the air conditioner. She found out why, when she overheard one of the men saying he knew when the blowers for the air conditioner went on because "Helen's nipples hardened right up."

Helen complained to her boss who laughed and said, "Boys will be boys. Besides," he continued, "it was just a practical joke. Where's your sense of humor?"

However, nobody laughed the day the air conditioner broke down. Hot, humid, and stale air pressed down all around them. Someone had "accidentally" spilled glue down onto the fans, causing the motor to lock up. It was nearly a week before the mechanics could get the glue off the blower blades. Helen's desk was returned to its previous position and no questions were asked concerning the subtle sabotage of the air conditioner. Helen felt she had the proverbial last laugh at the "boys' " expense for a change.

* * *

It was just before five when Carol returned Helen's call. Helen explained Nicole's situation. Carol was silent as she digested the information.

"That bastard," she finally uttered. "He's still at it. When I think of what he did to me, I still get furious. How's Nicole handling it?"

"Not well," replied Helen. "She can't believe it is happening to her. She's angry at him, and she blames herself. The sad part is she really thought highly of this jerk, and wanted to learn from him. I invited her to our lunch date tomorrow. Is that okay with you?"

"Yes, of course." Carol paused. "I know I did the right thing at the time, but I wish I could have taken him on when he harassed me."

"You did what was best for you," stated Helen. "Don't forget the price you paid. You should be president of a company right now, not just one of the vice-presidents. He set your career back 5 years. If not for your determination and stamina, it could have been much longer. He came close to destroying your career completely."

"Yeah, but look at what's happening now. If I had confronted him back then and filed a formal complaint, instead of leaving the company, Nicole wouldn't be faced with the same no-win situation. At least, he would have thought really hard before pulling this crap again."

"Carol, we've gone over this before. You made your decision. It was the right one at the time. Remember what Pam, in accounting, had to do about her problem?"

"I'm not sure I remember . . . ?"

"Sure you do. Pam had this one jerk staying late in the office anytime she worked late. Everybody else in the office had gone home and . . ."

"Oh, yeah, now I remember. He would fake like he didn't know she was still there and unbuckle his pants, let them drop to his ankles and then he'd start to scratch himself. At first Pam thought he didn't know she was there. She didn't want to embarrass him so she kept as quiet as she could until he left."

"Yeah," continued Helen, "but she caught on when it happened again. She was positive he knew she was still in the office. Finally, he did it where she had to see him, and he had to see her. Pam said, he didn't even try to act surprised to see her."

"I thought she handled that pretty well." Carol chuckled.

"Perfectly." Helen laughed. "I mean the fool even waved when she took his picture. She had a hard time keeping herself from bursting out in laughter, as he shuffled over to her desk with his pants around his ankles, only to see her drop the picture into an envelope already addressed to his boss. She put it in her locked drawer and told him it would stay there, as long as he didn't pull that stunt again."

"And he didn't," declared Carol. "Of course, it doesn't always go that smoothly," Carol added with a serious tone to her voice.

Carol abruptly changed the topic. "Nicole is going to have a harder time. This isn't a coworker. This is her boss. The same man who, when he was my supervisor, felt he had the right to let his hands roam over my body."

"You confronted him," interjected Helen. "You threatened to report the incident to his boss."

"Yeah, and what did he say? He said 'It was just an office thing. A natural occurrence when males and females work closely together.' He knew full well I would be ending my career if I reported him. I would have been ostracized. He would have received a lecture from his boss and I'm the one that would have been transferred or fired. Look what happened to that newscaster in Buffalo, Kathleen Neville.[1] She was in legal battles for something like 10 years. And she never did get her job back. It totally ruined her career in broadcasting. On the one hand, I'm glad I chose to leave the company, but I've never been completely happy with my decision to leave."

"It was right for you. You survived. You salvaged your career," reasoned Helen.

"Yes. Maybe you're right. It still doesn't seem fair. When is that company going to wake up and realize it is losing a lot of excellent employees? Look at the number of people who left after what happened to me. It was common knowledge, and they did nothing to discipline him. Joe Trackman left because he didn't like the signal it sent to the rest of the employees. Lisa Giddeon transferred out of the department, and subsequently left the company. They're both working for the competition now. And they're not alone, others have left, too. Do they value their employees so little? When for God's sake will they . . ."—Carol quit talking for a second, then continued—"Helen, you're supposed to stop me when I start ranting and raving like this."

"I know. Maybe I let you go on because I'm so upset about Nicole. Anyways, let's discuss this tomorrow. Blue Spruce Cafe at 1:30. I'll bring Nicole."

* * *

"It all seems like a dream today," apologized Nicole, as she slid into the booth at the Blue Spruce. "I'm sorry for overreacting. I feel kind of foolish. I'm sure he meant nothing by what he said. As you suggested, I went home yesterday and wrote down everything that happened, and exactly what he said. I read it over this morning. It all reads so harmless. Yet, at the time . . ."

Nicole reached for her glass of water and took a sip. An almost imperceptible shudder traveled up her back.

---

[1]Kathleen Neville's story is detailed in *Corporate Attractions: An Inside Account of Sexual Harassment With the New Rules for Men and Women on the Job* by Kathleen Neville, 1990, Washington, DC: Acropolis Books.

"I still feel his hands on my shoulders." She looked up. "Oh, Helen, I don't know what to think. I don't know how I can go back to work on Monday."

"You must go back to work Monday," implored Helen. She reached for Nicole's hand. "It isn't right for you to be the victim of his offensive behavior. You do have some options. We could discuss them if you want to."

Nicole released Helen's hand. She picked up her car keys and twisted them in her hands. "He's the boss. How can I fight him? If I report him he'll just deny it. It will be my word against his word. You know what that means. I'll be on the street looking for a new job without any references. Without references I'm sunk. I haven't made enough contacts in the field to overcome that." Nicole continued to fidget with her car keys.

Helen gave Nicole a worried look.

It was then that Carol walked up to the table.

"Sorry I'm late. I stopped by my office to pick this up." Carol held up a white envelope, addressed and stamped, but not sealed. "I thought I might show this to Nicole later."

"We haven't ordered yet," said Helen getting up and giving Carol a hug. "Carol, this is Nicole."

Carol shook her hand, and reached over with her other hand to give Nicole a comforting squeeze on her upper arm. "Helen has told me you have been initiated, by Mr. Powers, into the seamier side of Hale and Hale. I've come down that road, and if there is anything I can do to help I will."

"Thanks." Nicole sighed. "I'm really confused by all of this. One part of me wants to pretend it never happened, just ignore it and it'll go away. But another part of me would like to slit his throat."

Carol sat down. "You can always pretend it never happened, but it did. Ignoring it won't make it go away." As Helen and Nicole sat down she continued, "And slitting his throat wouldn't be a good career move. He'll never give you a good reference after that."

Helen and Nicole laughed out loud. Helen thought it was good to see Nicole relax and she was glad she had introduced the two women. They were still chuckling when the waitress came over to take their order.

Carol looked over the menu, proclaimed she deserved a good lunch because she skipped breakfast, and ordered the lunch special with a cup of soup. Helen settled for the lo-cal special saying she was saving herself for the creamy cheesecake for dessert. Nicole, after looking quickly at the menu, ordered a cup of soup and coffee.

"Did you have anything for breakfast?" questioned a concerned Helen.

"Coffee, and I made some toast. But it got cold before I ate it, and I threw it away. I haven't had much of an appetite lately," replied Nicole.

Helen and Carol exchanged glances.

"Nicole," started Carol, "I am really sorry this happened to you. I feel it is partly my fault."

Carol went on to reveal to Nicole her experiences with Mr. Powers.

"I think if I had confronted him then, you wouldn't be faced with this situation today," finished Carol.

"Thank you for telling me all of that," said Nicole, somewhat relieved. "I never dreamed anything like this would happen to me in the business world. I heard some stories of sexual harassment, but I just assumed," and here she gave Carol a guilty shrug, "that the woman who claimed sexual harassment was just angry at the man for a failed relationship. It was a way for her to get even. That's why at first I could only blame myself. But after listening to your story I feel more confident that it wasn't something I did."

"I am glad to see you're getting past the guilty stage," counseled Carol. "I felt that way the first time I experienced sexual harassment. I kept on trying to change whatever I was doing to cause it, but the harassment kept on happening. Once I decided it wasn't me, it didn't make it any easier to take, but at least I felt better about myself. I found I could then actively respond to the harassment instead of passively accepting it."

"I had a friend in college," said Nicole. "She was in the doctorate program while I was going for my master's degree. I found myself thinking about her last night. You see, she had an incident with her advisor, a well-respected professor in the field. He was married, but that didn't stop him from coming on to her. After class, in the middle of a philosophical discussion they were having, he made a comment about her eyes. At first, she was kind of pleased. She thought it was only some harmless flirting. She later told me she felt honored for the opportunity to have some excellent theoretical discussions with him. Well, something else happened. I still don't know what. There were rumors about allegations she made about him to the dean. At the time they had a policy of conducting all inquiries behind closed doors. Some settlement was reached. She wasn't allowed to discuss it. He continued teaching and she picked a new advisor. She ended up dropping out of the program a year later. I never really connected the two together."

Nicole looked at Helen and Carol. "That didn't have much to do with your comment, did it, Helen? I'm still not making much sense, am I?"

Helen patted Nicole on the hand. "You're making a whole lot of sense. Just keep talking about it."

"Now, I suppose it is my turn," Nicole said with a faint smile. "What do I do? Do I just drop out, fade away, or do I challenge him?"

"Times have changed," ruminated Carol. "You choices are much different from the ones I had. It seems like since the Anita Hill/Clarence Thomas thing, more women are speaking out about the sexual harassment they are experiencing. More companies are taking a proactive stance trying to prevent the occurrences of sexual harassment. I think Hale and Hale finally has a policy about what to do in the event a person experiences sexual harassment. Don't they, Helen?"

"Yeah," Helen smirked. "They brought in a consulting team to do a review of the personnel policies in place. It was rumored that they even received reports of possible sexual harassment cases. They then made recommendations on how to improve the procedure for reporting any occurrences. Nobody, other than the top executives, has seen the report. A memo was sent to all departments that there will be no sexual harassment tolerated at Hale and Hale. If an employee feels she or he has been sexually harassed they should report it to their supervisor." Helen looked at Nicole. "I don't think that policy is going to help you. Your supervisor is counting on his boss, Mr. Powers, to give him a favorable review and a recommendation for a promotion to head the new office that Hale and Hale is opening in Cincinnati."

"Maybe it is time I show you this," said Carol, as she pulled out the envelope she had brought with her. "I'm not sure it will help you in your decision, but it has helped me deal with the problem of sexual harassment and sexism."

Carol showed Nicole that the envelope was addressed to the president of the firm where Carol works. Carol pulled out the letter that was in the envelope.

"It is a letter that I wrote after working at the firm for 1 year. Each year I update it. Each year I have sworn I will send it. It is a letter that states that sexism and sexual harassment is damaging our firm. I recount actual cases of subtle sexism, accounts of sexual harassment inflicted on some of our brightest employees, who left because of it." She paused and looked at Helen before continuing. "I accused Hale and Hale of being insensitive to their employees, but it is a problem within my company also. In this letter I make a strong case for the elimination of these practices based on a zero tolerance policy that needs to be endorsed and followed by upper management. I recommend an educational program for all employees on male and female working relationships, similar in concept to other training programs we have. I've even written the outline for this educational program with its stated goals.

"I have to admit, the contents and the tone of this letter have changed over the years, as I have changed. I am now a vice-president of this firm. I have decided it is time I follow through on a belief I had early on in my life: that one person can make a difference. I've decided to send this letter."

Carol folded the letter and placed it back in the envelope. She held it in front of her, flashed Nicole and Helen a broad smile, and licked the envelope. Still smiling, she sealed it. "Well, let's go for a walk," she said.

Looking at Nicole, she added, "I have a letter to mail and you have a decision to make."

ACKNOWLEDGMENTS

The stories presented in this case study have been collected from a variety of sources, including media accounts, interviews from published research, and personal anecdotes conveyed to us. Thus, the main narrative is a fiction based on true accounts with slight alterations to protect the privacy of the "targets," "victims," and "survivors" of sexual harassment. The authors wish to acknowledge Doug Turner, Sib Law, and Tom Battaglia for their helpful criticism.

RELEVANT CONCEPTS

discursive practices
power imbalances
sexual harassment
societal attitudes
targets, victims, survivors

DISCUSSION QUESTIONS

1. Nicole seems to have a great deal of difficulty trying to describe the situation she encountered with Mr. Powers. What relationship exists between feeling like a "victim" and the ability to "name" and explain our experiences?

2. When Helen thinks back to the time that she was sexually harassed, she remembers how she put glue in the air conditioner. Can this act of sabotage be considered a discursive practice? Does this form of retaliation make management the "victim" of Helen's response?

3. Carol suggests that the letter she has written has changed over the years. How has Carol's image of herself changed in terms of whether she defines herself as a "target," "victim," or "survivor" of sexual harassment?

4. Nicole remembers a discussion in class where students debated the role of clothing in contributing to a woman's sexual harassment. In addition to clothes, what cultural artifacts contribute to labeling some individuals (male and female) as "targets" of sexual harassment? What cultural artifacts

contribute to blaming the "victim"? Does our culture signal a "survivor" of sexual harassment in any symbolic way?

SUGGESTED READINGS

Bingham, S. G., & Burleson, B. R. (1989). Multiple effects of messages with multiple goals: Some perceived outcomes of responses to sexual harassment. *Human Communication Research, 16*, 184–215.

Clair, R. P. (1993). The use of framing devices to sequester organizational narratives: Hegemony and harassment. *Communication Monographs, 60*, 113–136.

Kreps, G. L. (Ed.). (1993). *Sexual harassment: Communication implications.* Cresskill, NJ: Hampton Press.

MacKinnon, C. (1979). *Sexual harassment of working women.* New Haven, CT: Yale University Press.

Reardon, K. (1993, March–April). The memo every woman keeps in her desk. *Harvard Business Review*, pp. 4–8.

Taylor, B., & Conrad, C. (1992). Narratives of sexual harassment: Organizational dimensions. *Journal of Applied Communication Research, 20*, 401–418.

Wood, J. T. (1992). Telling our stories: Narratives as a basis for theorizing sexual harassment. *Journal of Applied Communication Research, 20*, 349–362.

PART IV

ISSUES RELATED TO HEALTH CONCERNS

13 *Without AIDS: A Gay Man Dies*

Frederick C. Corey
Arizona State University

Six days after our third anniversary, my partner was diagnosed with cancer. Eighteen days later he died. Kim's death reorganized my entire life. My being gay, once an immobilized position of shame, marginalization, and disenfranchisement, is now a point of political departure. In writing this essay, my aim is to present in narrative form the liminality between silence and speech, between privacy and public discourse; and I situate the limen in the context of communication about health, sexuality, and, ultimately, death. I address issues of patient–physician power, family communication, and the conterminous construction of gay men and HIV disease.

PHYSICIAN, PATIENT, AND THE NEGOTIATION OF POWER

In October 1990, while Kim was doing sit-ups, he hurt his rib. It appeared to be fractured, and he started a sequence of visits to physicians and chiropractors. After 2 months of these visits, I was sick of Kim being sick. I was tired of taking him to the medical offices. I was tired of going to the emergency room. I disliked hearing him moan. The pained look on his face got old. When I would ask what the physician said, he would reply with one word, "Nothing." This is ridiculous, I said, I am going to write a letter to the physician. And so I did:

December 1, 1990

Dear Dr. Fine,

I am writing to you about Kim Bauley, a patient in your office. Kim and I are relational partners, and though he does not know the exact content of this letter, he does know that I am contacting you.

We are not satisfied with his rate of recovery. As you know, on October 19, 1990, Kim was doing sit-ups and he fractured his rib. This was diagnosed almost immediately, and he was led to believe it would heal on its own within a couple of weeks. He has not recovered; on the contrary, his pain seems to be worse than ever, and even the slightest amount of movement increases the pain dramatically.

Three problems beyond the rib have made themselves apparent. First, he has trouble breathing. This problem comes and goes, and though it is not as bad now as it was around November 17, we are worried that his trouble breathing could return at any time, and should this trouble return, we do not know what to do, except perhaps to call you.

The second problem is more immediate. Kim has been constipated since around November 19. On November 28, at 11:30 p.m., he was in excruciating pain, for he was trying to defecate but could not—the feces was like a large rock lodged in his orifice. I took him to the emergency room at Scottsdale Memorial where they gave him an enema and said that this was not unusual for a person taking Tylenol Three. He is still not having normal, healthy bowel movements.

The third problem is more mysterious, and it concerns his liver. He is having tests done on his liver, but he does not seem to have good information regarding the nature of the tests. What exactly is being tested? He shared a drinking glass with a friend who has Hepatitis B last month—should we be worried about Hepatitis?

Four problems, then, are in need of attention: a fractured rib, trouble breathing, constipation, and an apparently symptomatic liver.

Dr. Fine, I am not unsympathetic to the pressures facing physicians. I have seen the effect of stress your occupation involves. I realize that you must have a number of patients with life-threatening or advanced stages of illnesses. I also realize, though, that proper early treatment and detection can reduce the onset of advanced problems.

Kim's problems have advanced. We would like to work with you to arrest the onset of new problems and resolve the problems which already exist.

I propose a change in procedures at two levels, the first rather general, and the second specific. The general procedures I suggest are as follows:

—If the medication administered has known side-effects, please let us know and tell us what to do should these side-effects occur. For example, if Tylenol Three causes constipation, is it okay to take a laxative with the Tylenol Three? I have discouraged him from taking oral laxatives because I know they can be toxic, but I don't know anything about medications. He seems to be urinating an awful lot—is there a type of diet that would divert the liquid to soften the feces?

—When you are conducting a battery of tests, please take the time to explain what is being tested and what might be revealed through the tests. When the test results are in, please explain them thoroughly.

—Please take the time to listen to Kim when he is trying to tell you what is going on inside him. He is not ill often, and he does not normally have aches and pains, so the vocabulary is foreign to him. I took him to an appointment in your office on November 19, and we arrived promptly at 10:00 and waited until 11:30, and then when you visited with him, you were in the examination room for less than five minutes. This is simply not reasonable. Very little communication can occur in a context that involves a 90-minute wait for a 5-minute contact. (I will point out that he is seeing a chiropractor, not because the chiropractor is administering great medical treatment, but rather because the chiropractor is explaining the nature of the fracture. This information should be coming from his primary care physician.)

The specific actions I suggest are:

—Kim needs to get a second opinion on his general condition, and this opinion should come from someone respected by both of you. Please recommend someone and help us get an appointment with that person within the next day or so. Perhaps an osteopath would be appropriate, given the overall nature of his problem.

—His medications need to be reassessed. The Tylenol Three appears to be hurting the proper functioning of his bowels, and there seems to be some suggestion that the anti-depressant drug is damaging the liver. (It is *not* helpful, though, to tell him on Friday that he should just stop taking all medications and then come in on Monday. This type of assessment serves to belittle the terrible pain he is enduring.)

Again, let me assure you that I am not oblivious to the demands of your profession, and I realize you cannot drop everything for a patient who just happens to wander into your office with a pain in his side.

I am hoping, though, that you will work with us to get Kim back on his feet. He is under a lot of stress that will not be going away. He had planned on starting design school effective December 3, and he quit his 12-year job in retail management to pursue that plan. Thinking that he would recover by December 3, he submitted his resignation in mid-November. December is here, but he is not well enough to be in school, so he is without a job, and he is not recovering.

Let me close by noting that I am a third party and the content of this letter is, to some extent, beyond my privilege. Kim feels, however, as many Americans feel, that if he asserts himself with the physician, the physician will provide less professional health care. Now, I know this is absurd, and you know this is absurd, but there's no persuading people on issues involving such high-level vulnerability.

Kim has always had an aversion to physicians, but he feels comfortable with you and he trusts your medical judgment. When he broke his arm, I had to drag him kicking and screaming to get it fixed—he wanted to let it heal on its own!

I appreciate his respect for and trust in you, and I am grateful.

Sincerely,
Frederick C. Corey

I slipped the letter through the wrought-iron gate protecting Dr. Fine's office and felt a pang of trepidation. Would the letter blow away? Would the custodian sweep the sealed envelope into the trash? Would the physician read the letter and find it presumptuous? I went home and told Kim about the letter. He did not ask to read a copy.

On Monday morning, Dr. Fine called. He wanted both of us to come in that afternoon. We arrived early and waited. I tried not to be irritated. The nurse opened the door and called our names, and she brought us into an examination room. I was surprised, for I expected to be shown into his office. I asked the nurse if Dr. Fine wanted to see us in an examination room or his office. She assured me we were in the proper room. I sat in a chair, and Kim sat on the examination bed, on the white paper that crinkles and crackles with every turn.

"Let me do the talking," I said to Kim.

"Just don't embarrass me," Kim said, and we both smiled because we knew I would. He looked scared.

Finally, the door opened. Kim was right. Dr. Fine was a handsome man, tall and tanned and confident. I stood and extended my hand. He shook it, apparently under duress, and gestured to the chair. I started to smile, a nervous habit, and I found myself looking up at him. Dr. Fine chose not to sit. "I have never received a letter like this," said Dr. Fine.

"First time for everything," I said. At first, I was not able to read his behavior, but he quickly clarified his overall response. He was furious. Kim and I exchanged nervous glances, and for a moment, I wanted to crawl into a hole and die. Dr. Fine stood over us and slapped the letter with the back of his hand. I sat in the chair and looked at my shoes.

I had dressed for power. I wore clothes that made me feel confident and aggressive. Burgundy loafers, woven socks, navy wool slacks with cuffs, burgundy belt, blue striped shirt, and a tie that was red with large, blue polka dots. I dressed carefully, prepared myself for the negotiation of power between patient and physician.

But I was trumped. Dr. Fine had all I had but more. The way we were positioned, when I looked straight ahead, I was at eye gaze with the cloaked source of his power. When I looked at the floor, I felt defeated. When I met his eyes, I felt beneath him, lower than his position in the hierarchy of the patriarchal pecking order. I was in a no-win situation. I sat in the chair while Dr. Fine used the social economy that was supposed to be on my side as a weapon against me. What was left in my hand was my great disadvantage: I am a fag. I felt powerless.

Or, to the contrary, was I placed within what Foucault (1976/1978) called a "manifold sexuality" (p. 47), a relationship invested with procedures of power? Foucault argued that with the advent of the classification of same-sex desire as "homosexuality," the temporary aberration of incidental sodomy became a human species infused with the power of curiosity and exclusivity. What was once an act that occurred between two people became a genre of human beings, and, from the perspective of medical science, these deviates needed "examination and insistent observation" (p. 44). That Kim and I were brought into the examination room was, from a Foucaultian perspective, no accident at all. Kim and I—two White men who appeared otherwise "normal"—needed to be inspected. Kim and I found ourselves in the examination room with the history of medicine. We found medicine "caressing them [us] with its eyes, intensifying areas, electrifying surfaces, dramatizing troubled moments" (Foucault, 1976/1978, p. 44). Three men in an examination room. Each is tall. Each is White. Each is well dressed. Each is attractive. Each has ego. One is dying. One is a physician. One wrote a letter. All three men in Foucault's examination room are "exercising a power that questions, monitors, watches, spies, searches out, palpates" (p. 45). We evade this power, fool it, and enjoy the pursuit. The scandal, resistance, capture, and seduction are pleasurable.

"I am a doctor," said Dr. Fine, "and I have patients who are dying. If you have to wait, you have to wait." I should have stood up, turned to Kim, and said there was not enough space in the examination room for a patient and this physician's ego. The immediate is not a retrospect, though, and the progression of crisis is incremental.

I sat silently, and Kim entered the panic mode. "I don't mind waiting," he said, and Dr. Fine was appeased.

"Is this all?" I asked, not knowing what I meant by the question. The power relationships were established. Kim and I were subject to the constraints and will of the physician, and, from his domain, we could proceed. The physician relaxed, leaned against a counter, and said, no, this (the exercise of power?) was not all, we should talk.

The textual meaning of our conversation was marked not by what we said, but instead by the amount of tension in the room, and over the next 30 minutes, the tension rose and fell. Dr. Fine set the tone by relaxing and talking to Kim for a few minutes. They liked each other, and I saw their rapport. The tension rose, though, when Dr. Fine turned to me to talk about the constipation. "Is it true," I asked, "that Tylenol Three causes constipation?"

"Not unless he has arthritis. Does he have arthritis?"

"Maybe," I said. "Maybe he does."

"Tylenol Three causes constipation in old people with arthritis." The doctor spoke.

The discussion made its way to AIDS and the HIV test. I had been tested for HIV when Kim and I started dating, and I was negative. Kim had never been tested. He was afraid. "We should get a test," Kim said to Fine. I said we would need to go to the county for an anonymous test, because what with Kim just quitting his job, he did not want to jeopardize his insurability. The physician agreed.

"But I want you to get tested," he said. Kim started to say something, but he stopped when the physician raised his eyebrows, as if to suggest AIDS was really the issue here. I said that I have worked at the local AIDS project for several years, I have seen plenty of AIDS cases, and what Kim had just did not look like AIDS.

"But I want you to get tested," he repeated. "And you should, too," he said to me.

"Let's suppose it's not AIDS," I said. "What do you really think it is?"

"Stress," said the physician.

"Stress?" asked Kim. He lit up for the first time in the examination room. He appeared relieved, hopeful.

"Yes," said Fine, "stress. How's school?"

"I haven't started yet," said Kim, and I refrained from noting that was in my letter. "I have been sick."

"Al Collins is a friend of mine," said Fine, "and—"

"He's not going to Al Col—" I interrupted.

"Well," Kim interrupted, "I might. I haven't decided."

I should have let it drop, but I could not thwart a look of aghast in plain view of the physician. "Where are you going to school?" asked Fine.

"I am going to interior design school," said Kim. "I just don't like the sound of interior design."

With perfect bedside manner, Dr. Fine asked Kim about interior design school and treated the topic without judgment. He and Kim again engaged in a jovial conversation about interior design. When they were through, everyone was in good spirits, relieved to believe Kim's problems were stress related and everything would be fine. As we were leaving, I asked about the second opinion, and the physician said we wouldn't need a second opinion. He'd run some more tests. "And you are going to the county. Right?"

I took the day off work, and Kim and I spent the entire afternoon at lunch, going to a movie, and shopping. It was one of my happiest days with Kim, because we were communicating at a level of honesty two people rarely achieve. We talked about feeling vulnerable in the examination room, being afraid of disease, and reducing stress in our lives. We found the power to be open in the context of the examination; the blush of vulnerability and strength of self-determination coexisted under the careful eye of medical science. "Power," wrote Foucault (1976/1978), "is not something that is acquired, seized, or shared, something that one holds on to or allows to slip away" (p. 94). When I dressed for power, I thought I would seize something. I mistakenly believed that the physician had something I wanted. I thought he had control over Kim's life. I thought he had information that would perpetuate living. I wanted to penetrate institutional organizations of power, at both superstructure and base levels, but instead, I found myself in agony.

Neither side was willing to give in completely. As Foucault posited, "power is exercised from innumerable points, in the interplay of nonegalitarian and mobile relations" (p. 94), and, in our situation, the triangulation of power in the examination room was in a constant state of flux. The physician was in his territory. The patient's body was the center of attention. And I deployed tactics of aggression and patients' "rights."

A patient has the right to secure a second opinion, and a physician has the right to know the HIV status of a patient. A patient has the right to background information on medications, and a physician has the right to set priorities. A patient has the right to be assertive, and a physician has the right to resent third-party interference. But rights are a moot point in physician–patient relationships. The communicative relationship between a physician and patient is established not in the realm of rights, but instead in the procedural negotiation of power. There is no escape from power, for it is omnipresent and located at base levels of interactions. The physician and patient deploy tactics and strategies that result in exchange and mobility; what may be a point of power at one moment becomes a source of default at the next, and what is a weakness outside the physician's office can be used as a point of power inside the office. It is valuable to note, too, that the base deployments of power are connected to superstructures of social power, but the superstructures, like base displays, are mobile and fluctuate between advantage and disadvantage. The grand scheme of institutionalized medicine carries with it a legacy of control and dominance, and the generic categorization of homosexuality as perversion is imbued with lack of control and repression. It would be unfair, though, and even incorrect, to say that it therefore follows that, at the base level, physicians deploy the history of medicine as an oppressive tool against sick homosexuals. One on one, the exchange of power becomes more complicated.

AIDS is one of the complications. Particularly for gay men, AIDS has produced ramifications that are economic, emotional, behavioral, social, cultural, and psychological. I speak here of the very obvious. We are afraid to quit our jobs for fear of losing our health insurance, for example, and we are drained from watching friends and acquaintances die. Our families and friends equate our bodies with illness, leading to formations of gay and lesbian communities that serve as surrogate families. We manage sexual risk or feel guilty when we take risks, or we act with reckless abandon. And when we are ill, we live with the fear, generated from internal and external sources, that we have HIV disease. A cold that will not go away creates an internal panic, "It must be AIDS." A pain in the side that defies explanation elicits the raised eyebrow from the physician, "Might there be a systemic problem?"

Today, it is possible to go to the local clinic, pay $75, take the AIDS test, and get the results in 3 hours. When Kim was sick, testing was not as expedient. The county clinic was backlogged, and we had to wait 2 weeks for the next available appointment, and then we would have to wait another week for the results. I was certain, when we left Dr. Fine's office, that Kim did not have HIV disease. He had none of the classic symptoms. Maybe it is stress, I said to myself, and maybe I am causing his stress, maybe the career change was my idea, not his. We made the appointments for both of us to be tested for HIV.

Two nights later, Kim had night sweats, a classic symptom of HIV infection. There was no denying that these were night sweats: The bed was drenched. While I was tossing the sheets into our brand-new washing machine—honestly, there was nothing wrong with the old one, but Kim said it was no good because it left lint on the black turtlenecks—I assured Kim that night sweats did not mean AIDS, that there were night sweats long before there was AIDS. Deep down, though, I thought, this is it. *It must be AIDS.*

Diagnosis and Hospitalization

On Wednesday, December 18, 1990, Kim had to go in for another test of some sort, and because his mother was in town, she would take him. I could spend the day at the office getting ready for the final exams I would be giving on Thursday. I was relieved—I had read every magazine in every physician's office in Scottsdale, and this would give Betty something useful to do.

I talked to Kim in the early afternoon. We did not say much, but then, around 5:30, he called me from the physician's office. He had to go to the hospital right away. I remember only three words—liver, bone, and cancer. I stopped thinking. I went home and went into the bathroom where I started to pack an overnight bag. I heard the front door open. Kim entered the bedroom, closed the door behind him, and said to me in a voice that could not have been more clear, more precise, more terrified: "I have cancer."

He started to cry. As I held him, I knew everything was changed. I began living on two simultaneous planes: the first, the survivor—the task-master, he who packs an overnight bag, remembers the toothpaste, an extra toothbrush, a list of phone numbers and the insurance card; the second plane, the knower—the sad one, he who now discovers everything will not be okay, will not be good, will not work out, no matter how much planning, trying, manipulating, or hoping; no matter how good things may seem, life is a tragedy punctuated by a few pleasant moments.

We drove to the hospital and checked Kim into a room, but he was assigned a double room, and the man in the next bed was surrounded by his wife and children. As we were fixing Kim's bed, he asked me if the hospital had private rooms. I said I would ask, and I went downstairs to admissions. I said to the clerk, "My lover has cancer, and he is in Room 521 West. Are there any private rooms?"

"Yes," said the clerk, "but your insurance won't pay the additional cost." She looked at me. When she told me the additional cost would be $30 a night, I said that would be fine, I would pay the additional cost. "Then," she said, "if I put an X in this little box right here, it won't cost you anything at all. There. There's an X in the box."

"Thank you. Thank you," I said. "You are very kind."

We moved to a private room and escaped omnipresent heterosexuality. We did not have to endure the glances, the stares, and the remarks. Best of all, we could live with complete disregard of visiting hours.

When Dr. Fine arrived at the hospital, he pulled me aside. "Did you get the test?" he asked.

"We are scheduled for tomorrow," I said.

"We will have to conduct the test here," he said. "Kim will have to sign this form." Fine took a piece of paper out of his file and showed it to me.

The form was a government document and resembled informed consent. The test results will be held confidential, it said, and "positive test results will be reported to state and local health authorities." As I read the form, I thought about how the American government does not protect a patient against discrimination based on real or perceived HIV status. This has since changed to some extent through the Americans With Disabilities Act, but in 1990, the people perceived to be HIV positive were subject to legal terrorization.

I asked Dr. Fine, "What if he refuses to sign this?"

"He has to sign it," said Fine.

"Do you see the irony?" I asked. "The results are confidential, but they are reported to the government. The results are protected by law. What law?" Dr. Fine looked at the form, as though for the very first time, and agreed that yes, the form is absurd, but he assured me he didn't write it, and the hospital required him to secure a signature. The form, for the physician, is a ritual prescribed by the government. Given the absence of substantial financial rewards, the physician has no motive to disobey governmental rules. Dr. Fine shrugged his shoulders. Kim signed the form. No one, it appeared, had any choice. We consigned reason, conscience, and responsibility to the anonymous power structure organized under the rubric of the department of health.

At Kim's request, I went shopping for pajamas, pure white, all cotton.

Family Matters

Christmas Eve became a day of family and death as a certainty. I woke up at 5:30. It was too early to go to the hospital—Kim usually woke up around 8:30—so I decided to write a letter to my parents and tell them everything. I told them I am gay, I had a lover, and he was sick. I viewed the letter as little more than a task, for in the context of Kim's illness, my biological family was of little consequence to me. I had no idea how my parents would respond to the letter.

I knew, though, that I had to deal with the Parent Problem. My brother Pat had been trying to reach me by phone, and when I would arrive home from the hospital, I would find messages like, "Call Pat immediately." I threw the slips of paper away. A couple of days later, Pat called very early in the morning. Thinking it was Kim, I answered. "Fred," he said, "you have to talk to Mom and Dad." I was the best man at Pat's wedding, and during the reception, my mother was in an excellent mood, holding the people at her table captive with her views on politics and the Catholic church. "I don't want to go to church," she said, "and hear the priest read a letter from the Bishop telling us how the Pope feels we should vote." She then railed on the Church's treatment of Geraldine Ferraro, on how based on the single issue of abortion we were to vote for Ronald Reagan. "Sexism," she said. "Nothing but sexism. The Church does not respect women. Never has. This has got to change." I liked my mother when I heard her talk like that, and I credit my ability to think independently to her, but I was deeply hurt when she concluded her views with, "Only one thing I agree with the Pope on, and that's the question of homosexuality."

She then turned to my brother Bob and asked him what he thought about the question, and I wondered why she was asking Bob. As though to garner support, she asked my most conservative brother, the one who says he likes his house but hates the neighbors, "especially," he said, "those two queers down the street. I don't understand it, and I think it's sick."

My father looked uncomfortable, and I wondered what he was thinking. I wondered if what I had heard was true, that he once said he'd rather his son were dead than gay. I felt small in my silence.

As I finished the letter, the phone rang. I went into the bedroom, picked up the receiver, and I heard Kim on the other end of the line, screeching. I screeched back. Finally, he told me what I already knew. The physicians said there was nothing they could do. He would be dead within a year.

I drove to the hospital and we sat together, silently. He asked me to tell his parents. I called Betty and John and told them that this would be a good time to come down to the hospital, and when they arrived, I brought them into a little waiting room. We all sat down, and I held John's hands as I said, loudly, for he was largely deaf, "Today, it's okay to cry." My relationship with Kim's family is a study in itself, more closely related to family studies than health communication. Betty and John are simple people from a small town in North Dakota, and it was difficult to determine what they were thinking or how much they knew. They were not strangers to me; they spent winters in Arizona, and they would stay with me and Kim.

They slept in the guest bedroom, and Kim and I maintained our normal routine. We shared the same clothes, wore matching rings, and slept together. Betty told her friends, "The boys are bunking up." At the hospital, the physicians, nurses, insurance agents, and administrators openly avoided Betty and John. Upon the agreement of all parties involved, I served as a liaison between the hospital and Kim's family. On occasion, John would interpret my role through a mumble, "Boy, he's some friend."

After I told Kim's parents the cancer was terminal, I left them alone and took my daily walk through the park next to Scottsdale Memorial. At the distant corner of the park is a magnificent sculpture by Louise Nevelson, and I walked around and around the sculpture, wailing faithfully, and, when through, I returned to the hospital. The mood was calm, and Dr. Fine arrived. He was somber as he talked about the cancer, but then he said, in a hopeful tone, "The AIDS test came back negative." He added, "We can run another one."

The Reemergence of AIDS

It Must Be AIDS. When a 35-year-old gay man has a terminal illness, it must be AIDS. A social equation exists between gay men, illness, and HIV disease. This equation, although based in the partial fact that HIV has high correlation to gay men in America, is actually one of convenience. AIDS provides quick and comforting explanations. *Convenience 1:* The mysterious illness, desultory symptoms, or bizarre bodily reactions to medications can be explained by contextualizing the gay man's body as a house of AIDS. *Convenience 2:* The tragedy of a young man dying can be shrouded in the stigma of AIDS, thereby reducing the tragedy through silence, the absence of explanation. *Convenience 3:* The physician is not responsible for trying to cure a gay man's sick body, for AIDS has no cure. And the most violent of all, *Convenience 4:* Whatever ails a gay man—HIV, hepatitis, herpes, syphilis, gonorrhea—is something he has brought upon himself. The physician is not responsible.

In reality, physicians are not responsible for any of their patients' illnesses, with the possible exception of some cases of malpractice. In our case, though, corrigible discourse, not malpractice, is the central concern. Kim's cancer was fatal regardless of the physician's talk about stress or the connection between gay men and HIV disease. The diagnosis could have been correct from the start, and Kim would still be dead. Nothing could have saved him from the cancer. What can be corrected is the violent discourse that connects gay men with AIDS, the rhetoric of the "not-innocent victim." Here we find ourselves immersed in the destructive social discourse surrounding AIDS. When we say, for example, that babies with

AIDS are "innocent victims," we imply that others (read: gay men) are guilty victims. The guilt is linguistically constructed through the default position, and the placement of guilt upon the person with the disease relieves the larger society from feeling guilty about the lack of medical attention given to HIV disease. That is, society does not need to feel guilty about the pain and suffering endured by people with AIDS because the patient, not the society, is guilty, and guilt, as it is constructed in our society, is not a shared commodity, but instead a verdict placed upon one party. The violence of this discourse, taken to its extreme, becomes played out in physician–patient relationships. Physicians do not like to see their patients suffer, and, as a general rule, physicians try to help their patients. When a patient is in chronic pain, however, and cures and treatments are futile, it is natural that the physician feels terrible.

The rhetoric of AIDS provides physicians with an escape from their discomfort. The patient is in constant pain, but whose fault is that? Gay men have brought AIDS upon themselves. I contend, then, that when Dr. Fine wants to conduct yet another test for HIV, he is acting in part to solve the mystery of the cancer, but in larger part, he is absolving himself of his "terrible feelings" over Kim's pain. The last time Dr. Fine mentioned the AIDS test was a few days before Kim died. We were walking down the hall of the hospital, talking about the quick progression of the cancer, and Dr. Fine said we could still do another test, we could even take blood from the corpse. "Would you knock it off with the AIDS stuff," I said sharply. "He does not have AIDS."

He stopped and looked surprised. "I am not used to seeing my patients die," he said. "I feel terrible."

"Well," I said, "get used to it. Watching people die is what a doctor does."

The next day, I received word to "lay off" Dr. Fine. This word came from a friend, an interior designer, who was helping Dr. Fine's wife redecorate their house. She said her husband felt just awful about Kim. Ironically, Dr. Fine had no reason to feel terrible about Kim's pain. He had no impact whatsoever on his patient's body.

CONCLUSION

Kim died on January 12, 1991. His parents never acknowledged the romantic relationship between me and Kim; we remained close, however, and after Kim's death, we spent time together daily. My own parents responded well to the letter I wrote on Christmas Eve, and they expressed compassion over the cancer. After Kim died, though, they tried to "normalize" our relationship by not talking about Kim dying or my being gay.

After a year of their normalizing strategies, I told them it is important I talk about being gay and losing a lover. They were unreceptive, and in a pivotal conversation with my mother, I explained to her that I make a clear distinction between my biological family and the family of friends I need and love. I had no dire need to be with my biological family, and for all practical purposes, I considered myself "divorced" from them. I was unwilling to compromise. I told my mother that either she accepts me for who I am, openly and without reservation, or we would no longer be in contact. She was jolted by my terms, but within a year she accepted them and she accepted me—on my terms. As a result, our relationship has strengthened. My mother now claims that her one great disappointment is that she never met Kim, and, she adds, "Whose fault is that?"

In this case study, issues of disenfranchisement are fluid rather than fixed. Marginalization involves negotiations of power, not categorical oppression. A gay White man with social privilege and good health insurance is not, by virtue of being gay, going to be ostracized by the medical industry. In the events surrounding Kim's death, the hospital staff was supportive and even generous. Encounters with the physician and family were more troubling. The physician did not like being told how to do his job. The physician covertly "examined" homosexuality, and he was reluctant to deconstruct the social equation between gay men and HIV disease. Kim's parents denied the relationship Kim and I shared, and my parents opted to make our relationship invisible. In sum, when confronting matters of physician–patient competition, denial, and invisibility, I have learned not to engage in a minoritizing logic of disenfranchisement and marginalization. Such a stance renders me powerless. Instead, I recognize the innumerable points from which power is deployed, and I begin processes of negotiation.

RELEVANT CONCEPTS

control over decision making
negotiation of power
social support
triadic communication

DISCUSSION QUESTIONS

1. Is it appropriate for a gay man's relational partner to write a letter to a physician about his partner's medical care? What are the cultural differences between a letter written by a heterosexual partner and a same-sex partner?

2. What led the gay couple to believe that their sexuality was being "examined" by the physician?

3. American culture creates a correlation between gay men and HIV disease. How does this affect medical care gay men receive?

4. Clinical tests for HIV antibodies are supposed to be held confidential but frequently are made public. How does the fear of disclosure impact communicative relationships between patients and their physicians, insurance companies, and employers?

5. From a communication perspective, what is the difference between a biological family and a family of friends?

6. Gay White men who come from privileged backgrounds are, simultaneously, members of society's most powerful class and among those most openly disliked or feared. How can gay men use verbal and nonverbal communication strategies to shift between these polarized positions?

REFERENCES/SUGGESTED READINGS

Crimp, D. (Ed.). (1988). *AIDS: Cultural analysis/cultural activism*. Cambridge, MA: MIT Press.

de Lauretis, T. (1991). Queer theory: Lesbian and gay sexualities. An introduction. *differences, 3*, iii–xviii.

Foucault, M. (1972). *The archaeology of knowledge/The discourse on language* (A. M. Sheridan Smith & R. Swyer, Trans.). New York: Pantheon.

Foucault, M. (1977). *Power/knowledge* (C. Gordon, L. Marshall, J. Mepham, & K. Soper, Trans.). New York: Pantheon.

Foucault, M. (1978). *The history of sexuality* (Vol. 1, R. Hurley, Trans.). New York: Random House. (Original work published 1976)

Foucault, M. (1982). The subject and power. *Critical Inquiry, 8*, 777–795.

Fuss, D. (Ed.). (1991). *Inside/out: Lesbian theories, gay theories*. New York: Routledge.

Warner, M. (Ed.). (1993). *Fear of a queer planet: Queer politics and social theory*. Minneapolis: University of Minnesota Press.

14 *Living With HIV and AIDS: Personal Accounts of Coping*

Sandra Metts
Heather Manns
Illinois State University

To write a case study of one person living with HIV or AIDS poses a serious challenge. Aside from the medical fact of being seropositive, these individuals are no more alike than any other group. They are members of every social community, ethnic background, and sexual orientation. Some become ill quickly and repeatedly, and face tremendous physical challenges; some experience very little physical change for many years. Some individuals are blessed with an accepting and supportive social network and some face the disease virtually alone. In short, the experience of each individual is unique. A typical experience or representative life story simply does not exist. For this reason, we have chosen to present here a composite picture, painted in broad strokes, of the experience of living with HIV and AIDS. We move through the "phases" from the time of the first diagnosis to the moments of reflection. We present the experiences of persons who shared their stories with us during extensive telephone interviews in the spring and summer of 1994. These 41 people, from around the United States and Canada, asked to be heard and we use this chapter to give them a voice.

OVERVIEW

Respondents

Respondents were alerted to the study through Internet bulletin board postings, announcements at support group meetings, and personal contacts. They made an initial contact with the authors via a 1-800 number obtained for the purpose of this study. Respondents were thereby able to leave a name (usually just a first name), a telephone number, and a convenient time for a return call with no expense to them personally. During the interview, we asked respondents to talk about the experience of being HIV positive or having AIDS, its impact on their professional, social, and personal lives, and any other issues that would "help social scientists better understand their experience." The only specific information sought was demographic information (e.g., age, state of health, employment, sexual orientation, gender, etc.), mechanisms for coping and avenues for social support, and effects on their relationships over the months or years since their diagnosis.[1] The length of the interviews ranged from 30 minutes to over 2 hours, with most lasting about an hour. Each conversation was transcribed by the author who conducted the interview.

After each interview, the authors discussed key issues that were evident in the interview. Particular attention was paid to issues that manifested one or more of the following features: (a) *repetition* (i.e., an informant returning to a concern, insight, problem, or consequence several times in the course of the interview), (b) *commonality* (an issue or concern that was raised by several respondents), (c) *intensity* (i.e., emotionally charged language or vocal tone), (d) *elaboration* (i.e., marked detail, description, and clarity of recall), and (e) *spontaneity* (i.e., issues raised with no prompting or expectation on the part of the interviewer). We considered these issues to be salient to respondents and allowed them to point us to themes that were worthy of note. In fact, the organization of this chapter was suggested by patterns in the interviews. Respondents frequently began their description of living with HIV and AIDS by taking the interviewer back to the time of diagnosis, or "discovery of infection" as it was often described. This date was for many a turning point marking a direction in life that cannot be reversed. Frequently this point of origin led to a discussion of how lovers (or spouses), friends, and family reacted to the news. These memories often led to discussions of depression and overcoming adversity, which led in turn to reflections on life since diagnosis. We have therefore divided this chapter into a loose chronology of three phases suggested by the interviews: discovery, relational consequences, and coping. In addition, several recommendations for future research were suggested by respondents. Thus, we conclude this chapter with specific concerns that persons living with HIV and AIDS would like to see addressed by social scientists working in this area.

---

[1]The sample was predominately White men. Four interviewees were women, five were African American, and two were Hispanic.

PHASES

Discovery

The statement, "You are HIV positive," changed the world for these 41 individuals. Needless to say, the circumstances of its telling were recalled with vivid clarity. In some cases, the message was not a surprise whereas in other cases it was.

It Was Inevitable. In the accounts of respondents who were *not* surprised by the diagnosis, a common theme emerged: "It was inevitable." For these individuals, a history of risky behavior, particularly IV drug use or unprotected sex, and/or the diagnosis of a sexual partner made the revelation of seropositivity an expected outcome. Carl's drug use, for example, led him to expect what he called "the logical end for a mixed-up life." He said of his experience:

> I lived on the streets in Chicago for 5 years. I got high every day. I think I would be dead right now if I hadn't gotten it [AIDS]. It was only a matter of time. I lived like an animal, on handouts and in homeless shelters. When I got sick, I went to the emergency room at Cook County and the doctor said, "We should do an AIDS test." I said, "Why bother? I can tell you right now that's what I've got." It was a no-brainer.

For many of the gay men in our sample who had been sexually promiscuous or engaged in unprotected intercourse prior to the AIDS outbreak, there was a sense of inevitability. As a number of respondents noted, members of the gay community assume every man they meet is HIV positive unless told otherwise. In fact, a very frequent comment made during the interviews was some variation of the statement, "It's not a matter of 'if' you'll get AIDS, it's a matter of 'when.' " For these men, chronic fatigue, weight loss, and persistent colds or flu were signs of what they already expected. As Allen recalled:

> In 1984 I started a new business in San Francisco. I was working 80-hour weeks with no time for myself. Then it really took off and so did I. I would have sex with two or three different men every night. I was getting rich and going crazy—free love and good times. I volunteered to have my blood frozen for the researchers who were developing the HIV test. Then in 1987 I got the flu and I couldn't shake it. My doctor tried everything. I told him about the blood sample and he called the clinic. Sure enough, I was HIV positive. I remember saying to the doctor that I was not surprised, that all my friends were in the same boat. Most are dead now. What surprises me I guess is

> that I am still here [small chuckle]. I smoke like a fiend and my doctor says I will die of lung cancer before I die of AIDS.

Allen's closing comment about his longevity is interesting. Increasingly, we became aware of a distinction implicit in many of the interviews between the HIV diagnosis and one's state of health. Respondents were clear that their HIV diagnosis was perceived to be inevitable, but this was not meant as a comment about the inevitability of bad health or death. Particularly for those respondents who had been HIV positive since the mid- and late 1980s, there were references to the fact that "in the early days" of the disease, the diagnosis was assumed to be the harbinger of death. But for those who were long-term survivors and for the individuals more recently diagnosed, the topic of the HIV diagnosis and matters of health were easily distinguished. As one respondent diagnosed within a year of the interview noted, "The doctors can all agree that you have it [HIV], but beyond that, no one knows if you'll live 1 year or 20 years. The results of the test are just that: the results of the test."

For some respondents, it was not their own health that signaled their HIV status, but the health of a sexual partner. For example, Joe noticed that his partner, Bobby, was getting weaker rather than stronger when they worked out in the gym. According to Joe:

> This man was a doctor of pharmacology and I felt that if anyone would know anything about their own health it would be him. He seemed to be ill most of the time but said it was nothing to worry about. When his parents came to visit they made him go to the hospital. He had had pneumonia for some time and said that he realized the first time he got sick that he had AIDS and he was afraid to tell me. So at that point I got tested and I was already at a low T-cell count. The relationship dissolved after that, but that was how I found out I was HIV positive.

When the relationship did not dissolve, respondents faced the double strain of dealing with their own diagnosis and tending to the needs of their partner. These needs are primarily physical (and medical) but often included the guilt of knowing they were responsible for infecting their partner. In Jay's words:

> John was fine with his own diagnosis, but he felt extreme guilt about mine. Because he was sickest first, he felt like he had given it to me. I put my heart and soul into caring for John and tried not ever to make him think I blamed him. After John died, all of those material things just didn't matter anymore.

Why Me? In some cases, receiving the news that one is HIV positive was totally unexpected. For these individuals, a common theme was "Why me?" During a routine physical for a job as a ranch hand in Arizona, Allen was told he was HIV positive. He recalled: "I was dumbfounded. I was straight, no drugs, no prostitutes. I went back for two more tests. It was true. I am still in shock."

For Margaret, a flight attendant based in Paris, the news was equally unexpected. She had a routine blood test as part of the preparations for her wedding. When the doctor called to tell her that she was HIV positive, she was sure she had simply misunderstood his English. She asked him to repeat his message in French, but the diagnosis was the same. According to Margaret:

> We went ahead with the wedding. It was a lovely ceremony but I was depressed. I felt like I should be wearing black instead of white. Everyone was somber. I'm okay with it now, but at the time I kept thinking, why me? My parents didn't know what to say and my husband's family thought it was something that would just go away. But the honeymoon was strained. We were afraid to talk about the future and about having a family. We stayed together for 3 years but we're separated now. He is on the fast track with his career and I want to stop and smell the roses.

Relational Consequences

As Margaret's experience indicates, the personal relationships of individuals who are diagnosed with HIV are directly and profoundly affected. However, we found that the effect was not uniformly negative. Although many respondents did describe the loss of family, friends, and lovers because of their HIV status, others told stories of remarkable loyalty and increased closeness. We turn now to several illustrations of each of these outcomes.

Rejection and Loss. For some respondents, disclosure of their HIV status resulted in the loss of a valued relationship. These losses were noteworthy to the respondents because they had not anticipated this outcome. Almost without exception, respondents commented that "some people will be put off by the fact that you are HIV positive or have AIDS, but 'true friends' will stand by you." What surprised respondents was when the reverse was true. That is, no respondent expressed surprise that coworkers, casual dating partners, distant relatives, and so on failed to support them. But several expressed surprise when coworkers and casual friends went to exceptional lengths to be supportive, whereas someone they trusted to stick by them failed to do so. William's experience illustrates this theme quite clearly:

> I was working as a psychologist in a family clinic in California. I put off telling my supervisor for months because I didn't know how she'd take it. Finally, I had to start taking time off for treatments and I had to tell her.

> You'll never believe what she did. She put out a memo asking all employees to contribute their vacation and sick leave days to my account. I got two full years of coverage out of that. Everyone was wonderful to me and my supervisor still calls to see how I am doing . . . But my lover at the time turned out to be a real disappointment. We were together for seven years and after I got tested he went in too. He was negative but said that he loved me and things would work out. Well after a few months, he got tired of me dealing with treatments and being sickly and he left. He just moved out one day, just moved out with half my stuff and left a note saying that he hoped I'd understand how he can't stay with me anymore and be around the illness. Well, I *didn't* understand and I still don't.

For several respondents, the loss involved a presumably close friend who abandoned the respondent. Both Jay and Lamont described their keen sense of loss and disappointment when a female friend let them down. Jay said:

> Melanie and I were like two peas in a pod. We did everything together. She even used to go to the gay bars with John and I. When I told her I was infected, she did not act like Melanie. Something about her had changed. She became a born-again Christian. Now my homosexual actions and lifestyle were wrong. . . . She was in my apartment only 20 minutes . . . she was the only person in the world who I thought would stand behind me, I was crushed.

Lamont echoed Jay's words:

> The two people I was closest to behaved very badly. One was a close female friend. She promised that she would take me to a hospital in Houston which was a three-hour drive. The hospital was offering a protocol. I mentioned the protocol odds, and the chance that it might not work anyway. She got very upset and said that it had to work and that she was going to take me there and make them put me on the drug. She never showed up that day to take me to the hospital. I guess she forgot what she said. My philosophy was that I would never call her again . . . People are very disappointing, changing their mind . . . relationships just weren't there, or at least they weren't as strong as I had assumed them to be.

Interestingly, later in the interview, Lamont mentioned this same trip to Houston but commented on the unexpected support received from his neighbors:

> Earlier I had mentioned that I was going to the protocol in Houston. And I remember he [a neighbor from Australia] had said "good luck" and I was very surprised. Then that morning when I left, his wife had said "good luck." So as I was on my way to the hospital, I stopped and leaned on the steering wheel and thought, what is this. I don't understand it. These people are just

> my neighbors and they wish me good luck. Of all the people I know and who I'm close to have not said anything and they just clam up and change the subject. This kind of brought up for me the issue of comfort. Who can comfort me? Who can hope for good news when it might be bad? I don't know what it takes exactly to do that, but it seems like a rare quality.

Some respondents expressed surprise and sorrow over the sense of being abandoned by their own family when they finally revealed their seropositivity. When Glen told his parents at the dinner table one Sunday, his mother began to cry and then left the room. His father said, "I hope you're happy now; you just broke your mother's heart." Glen's parents have not spoken to him in the year since his revelation. He commented on his disappointment: "I had been a model son, everything my parents wanted me to be and now I am some kind of piranha and they won't even set foot in my house." Bob experienced similar rejection by his family:

> I went to visit my brother during Easter vacation. He panicked when I told him . . . On Easter he went to his wife's family's house for dinner but didn't want me to go because he said they wouldn't understand. I spent Easter Sunday in a movie theater alone. And when I told my mom I was HIV positive she said that it was about time [because I am gay]. She sees AIDS as a punishment for my lifestyle.

Support and Confirmation. As indicated previously, our respondents also wanted to share experiences where support exceeded expectations. In these cases, personal relationships intensified. In the words of one respondent about his partner, "we stripped away all of the pretense and got down the essentials of living." This same respondent said of his partner:

> I keep telling him that he should leave and move on with his life. But he won't hear of it. He supports me financially and emotionally. He is with me every moment he is not at work. He does most of the cooking and all of the cleaning because my neuropathy has gotten so bad. He even bought me a puppy a few months ago. When I said I probably wouldn't be around to see it grow up he said, "cut it out" . . . I cough a lot at night and Jim sleeps upstairs. But he always gets in bed with me for awhile at night and we talk and he strokes me and then when I fall asleep he goes up to his own room. Can you beat that?

Parents and family also exceeded expectations. Of particular surprise seemed to be fathers. As Margaret noted, "My dad is the one who really surprises me. He used to sort of ignore me and now he even goes shopping with me [laughs] and even bought me a red convertible." Although Bob's own family was not supportive, he was struck by the support his friend received from his family. He said:

> I have a friend from Orlando. He is gay and HIV positive and his sister is straight and she is also HIV positive. Their parents are wonderful. The parents took the sister in to live with them. They offered to come and get him but he wanted to stay in California. But any time he is sick or needs something, his mom is on a flight to see him. Those parents give their kids such support and love.

And finally, from Mark who had kept a detailed diary of his life over the 6 years since his diagnosis, came this story:

> I knew I had to tell my family. My brother was getting married and I had to go back east for the wedding. I told my mother over the phone and she said she would tell my father. We had a plan that if he wanted to disown me, she would just tell people that something had come up and I couldn't make the wedding. I am the oldest son and my dad didn't even know I was gay. When I arrived, I was stunned. There was a big banner across the house that said "Welcome home Mark." They all treated me like a king and so did the whole wedding party. Now that I am too sick to travel my parents come out to California every couple of months and spend time with me. When my mom went to Disneyland the last time, my father stayed home with me because he said he just enjoyed our visits. If I hadn't been lying down, I would have fallen over.

Coping

Coping is the process of managing stressful events or circumstances that a person considers to be relevant to his or her well-being, but that strain or even exceed his or her resources (Lazarus & Folkman, 1984). Coping generally involves efforts to control stress through problem-solving strategies whenever possible, or through emotion-regulating strategies when the cause of the stress cannot be controlled.

During the course of the interviews, we realized that the coping process was remarkably individualized. The differences were due primarily to the fact that our sample of respondents was varied in terms of physical impairment and degree of network support. As a general claim, however, we can say that problem-solving approaches tended to deal with routine matters of work, health, and dating. Emotion-regulating strategies tended to focus on overcoming anger and depression.

Problem-Solving Strategies. For those respondents who were healthy and displayed no visible signs of illness, their life continued much as it had prior to their diagnosis. They went to work, paid bills, ordered pizza, and went to movies. These respondents described daily life as perhaps more "intense" and "appreciated" than before, and some were more attentive to living a healthier lifestyle, but in general they wanted us to know that they were living a "normal" life overall. We found, however, that even among this group, there were issues that required some degree of attention, if not strictly speaking, coping. These were often referred to as inconveniences or irritations. But we discuss them here as an aspect of coping because they required the psychological attention of the respondent and if not attended to, they became sources of stress.

One of the most common "inconveniences" was the need to remain healthy. Several respondents commented on the vigilance required to avoid opportunistic infections, for example avoiding people at work who had the flu, getting more rest than usual, and taking vitamins religiously. Other respondents commented on the need to change their lifestyle, especially employment and schooling. For example, Joe avoided giving up his job for as long as he could because he hated the thought of being on disability. "But," he said, "it was worth it; the amount of stress I've saved myself is unmeasurable. The secret is to know where your stress lies and to get rid of it. That's why I'm much healthier than others with the same T-cell count." And Lyle said, "The first thing I did was to quit school. It seemed silly to pursue a dream that I might not live to achieve. Now I have more time to relax." These were typical problem-solving techniques that helped respondents control stress related to their seropositivity.

A second common problem, less easily solved, was what to do about dating. The prospect of forming a serious relationship was problematic for those who had an active social life. Many respondents said that it was an "approach–avoid" issue because on one hand they desired the intimacy and on the other they couldn't face the pain of being rejected or watching a loved one die. Margaret, for example, commented on a recent party she attended where an attractive man asked her out. She declined the invitation, much to her regret, because she said, "There's no point in letting someone fall in love with a 'me' that will inevitably deteriorate." Margaret avoided the stress of dating by choosing not to date. Instead, she became active in public service. She became a public speaker at high schools, colleges, and civic groups to share her experiences and encourage young people to practice safer sex.

John too was concerned about future relationships:

> I am caught in a weird place. I don't want to fall in love with someone who is HIV negative because I might infect him or he might desert me when I get sick, but I don't want to have to nurse an HIV-positive guy while I still have my looks and my energy.

John's mechanism for coping with his dilemma was to build a social network over the Internet and go out socially with platonic friends.

For respondents who were experiencing signs of ill health, coping was more difficult. The intrusive effects of various protocols and treatment regimes complicated their lives in numerous ways. Again, dating seemed to be an arena of special concern. Matt, a self-avowed optimist, told us that he could find a way to laugh at just about anything but he had to admit that the side-effects of some treatments were starting to depress him. He observed:

> It isn't the physical pain, but the chipping away at your manhood, or personhood for that matter. I had to break a date three times with the same person because I got diarrhea so bad from a new medication that I couldn't be away from the bathroom for more than 15 minutes at a time. How embarrassing to have to say, "I can't go out, I'm still potty training." Getting an erection was clearly out of the picture.

Matt said he refused to stop dating but learned to cope with his limitations by dating only other HIV-positive men. As he explained his strategy:

> If I am not sure, I ask him right out whether he is positive or negative. If he says "negative" I walk away. But if he says "positive," then I know I have met a kindred spirit, I know he will understand the beauty of the good days and the ugliness of the bad days.

As Matt's comment indicates, the distinction between problem-solving and emotion-regulating strategies is easier to draw theoretically than pragmatically. Implicit in his decision to date only HIV-positive men (and in Margaret's decision not to date at all) was the desire to regulate emotional strain *before* it became a problem. However, for those respondents who did experience strong negative emotions, especially depression and anger, many relied on their own inner strength as a coping mechanism. Others relied on social networks for support and comfort.

Emotion-Regulating Strategies. For the most part, our respondents were comfortable with their lives and optimistic about the future. This was true even for those who were no longer able to drive because of neuropathy or poor vision, and those who were confined to bed for much of the day. In fact, we were struck repeatedly by responses to a closed-ended item regarding health that we had included among the demographic questions. On a five-point scale, with five representing "excellent health," the lowest score given was a three. This was offered by a man who was too weak to leave his bed and did much of the interview while he was on oxygen. His comment was, "I guess I would say a three; I'm doing pretty good these days."

This is not to say, of course, that our respondents did not face tremendous emotional challenges. Most respondents had experienced some degree of depression and anger, and the memories were vivid. Indeed, it appears that for many, the experience of feeling completely helpless and hopeless, hitting "rock bottom," as it were, served as a motivating force enabling them to get control of their lives and cope more productively. These periods seemed to come at certain points that were fairly common across respondents, particularly, (a) when first diagnosed, (b) when initial reactions from friends or family were not supportive, (c) when the respondent had to quit his or her job, or (d) when a close other died of AIDS (or committed suicide).

Sam's experience illustrates the depression that often accompanied the period of time around the initial diagnosis of HIV:

> A year before I was tested, I dwelled in negativity . . . for many years after I didn't want to make plans. I interacted less socially with other people. Currently I've developed more friendships and I've resolved to start dating again. But it took hitting bottom to bring me back out and to get involved again.

Daryl's depression occurred after he lost his job as a computer salesman (where a coworker tried to choke him when he revealed his seropositivity). Daryl said of his experience:

> I was so depressed that I sat in my apartment for weeks, barely eating or sleeping. I didn't answer the phone, I didn't call anyone, I just wanted to be completely alone. Then I realized that I was letting myself die before I was ready. I cleaned up one day and took myself to lunch. I had to hit bottom before I could start moving up again. I now do desktop publishing out of my apartment and I enjoy life again.

For Lamont, the negative reaction and withdrawal of his friends when he began to show signs of the disease prompted great anger. He said:

> I went through a period of one month where I got so angry that I decided that I wasn't going to call them, I was going to wait for them to call me. I'm embarrassed to say this but I stayed in bed for the whole month. I'd look at the phone all the time being so angry that no one had called. And after that month, after that 30 days I said to myself, I will never waste another month of my life like this. If they're not going to call, then I don't care. I'm still alive. I think I thought that I would die if no one cared. And so that month went by and I got out of the bed and I haven't stopped since . . .

For Sam, depression was associated with the death of his lover, Steven. Part of the depression was founded in the loss of a valued intimate, and some in the knowledge that he would eventually follow a similar path. According to Dan:

> When Steven and I had gotten together 12 years ago, we had made plans to build a home, etc. When you make plans with somebody—Steven was 34 when he died—I felt that all of my dreams had died with him. At that time I was concerned about when I would die, and at that time in history, people didn't make that much separation between being HIV positive and having AIDS. When Steven got very ill, I would wonder when I would also get sick. I was scared that I would be alone and I got very depressed.

For Ben, the anniversary of his friend's death tends to bring on depression. Part of the sorrow for Ben was that he assisted in the suicide:

> Like May 23rd is the suicide of my best friend here in the city. When I moved into my apartment building a few years ago, one of the first people I met was Mike. He committed suicide and I helped him—assisted with the suicide. And that's coming up and I'm trying to deal with that and there's a flood of memories and I still live in that same building.

Loss of self-esteem was also a major contributor to periods of depression. As scholars have noted, and individuals have experienced firsthand, AIDS carries with it a stigma more pronounced than any other illness. As Henry described the effect that AIDS had on his life he noted:

> It takes away your self-esteem, and you feel like contaminated property. You don't want to expose your emotions to other people and you don't want to get involved in a relationship. You don't want the person there while you go through the deterioration period . . . In a way I feel kind of like it puts your life on pause; you just stagnate . . . It takes away your self-worth and you feel like damaged goods. When you start feeling ill, it contributes to the problem of low self-esteem and makes it even worse. This is what leads to the depression, your lack of self-esteem.

Our respondents reported a wide range of emotion-regulating coping mechanisms. As might be expected, most relied heavily on support groups, friends, other HIV-positive individuals, therapists, and ministers or rabbis. For example, Bob identified his rabbi as a role model for his own self-discipline. He said, "My rabbi helps me to keep my sanity. Out of all my acquaintances, he is the best. He is my inspiration." For Richard, it was his partner who lifted his spirits: "When I'm depressed I turn to my lover. He makes fun of me. Usually when I'm depressed it's never what I think it's about, so he makes me laugh and I get out of it." For Carl, it was his support group, particularly his AA group:

> I like going to AA more than to the HIV support groups. At the AA meetings we talk about giving over to a higher power, about forgiveness, and taking life one-day-at-a-time. At the HIV meetings I hear guys talking about sex and bath houses and frankly that doesn't help me cope.

In addition to finding solace, comfort, and tangible assistance in the support network, some respondents found their own version of internal strength as well. For some, this strength came from religious reflection or inspirational reading. Paul read the Bible daily, Brad read Shakespeare and listened to classical music.

Others struggled with it on their own. Joe said that he copes with depression through denial: "Typically, I deny it as much as I can. At some point, reality does come crashing down on you. I rationalize reality when denial fails me. I say there are worse situations than mine."

Other respondents chose acceptance rather than denial. Michael's attitude, though more carefully articulated than most, is typical of the "resignation with purpose" theme that we observed in many of the interviews. Michael's explanation was triggered by an event at work when he complained of fatigue from working part time there and full time at another job:

> I can't stand it when they [coworkers] look at me and say "you're young, you can handle it" [working two jobs]. So I've told two people cause I was tired of them telling me over and over that I'm young and healthy. They were astonished. This one lady said, "Oh, I'm sorry and I wish it wasn't true." But I said, "I don't know if I wish it wasn't true; it's just a fact of life." She kept saying, "Don't you worry about it?" And I said, "No, I don't worry about dumb things anymore, I worry about kids who can't read or people without a home who can't find a job. I don't worry about myself because it's going to happen and I can't change that, but whatever's going to happen to those other people, I can change." There's nothing I can do about my homosexuality. There's nothing I can do about being HIV positive, but there are things I can do about other people's conditions. I can teach someone to read or I can help someone to find a job.

RECOMMENDATIONS

We asked at the close of the interview if there was any particular recommendation that the respondent could offer researchers that would lead to a better understanding of the experiences of living with HIV and AIDS. Many respondents said, quite simply, "Keep writing our stories."

Other respondents said they hoped greater effort would be directed toward educating the general public about HIV- and AIDS-related issues. In particular, respondents found their productivity and general quality of life diminished by the ignorance of other people, manifested in fear of contracting the virus through casual contact or proximity, or manifested in the assumption that death was imminent. As one respondent said:

> I appreciate people being sensitive to the fact that I have to take it easy sometimes, but I resent the hell out of people treating me like a freak. Publish something that tells them how to act toward me as a human being who has a virus, nothing more.

Two other issues were raised that were not common, but merit reporting. One issue was mentioned by a few of the homosexual men who were still sexually active. They advised concerted effort to understand the tremendous burden that HIV-positive men carried in terms of sexual responsibility. Several of these men said that they were trying to be very conscientious in their sexual relationships, but found that it was difficult year after year to be the "moral voice" in every encounter they had. As James explained the problem:

> I am an adult male with a PhD. I know what I have to do to protect my partners. But they say things to me like, "I don't care that you are positive; I don't want to use a condom and it's my decision to be at risk." I go into my spiel about my moral obligation, but you know, sometimes I get really tired of being my brother's keeper. As more and more of us live longer and longer someone will have to recognize the fact that a few PAs [public service announcements] will do little to change the reality of temptation during sex.

Although other respondents were less articulate than James, they too expressed the fear that they simply did not have the strength of character to maintain abstinence for the rest of their lives or to insist on the use of condoms during every sexual encounter. Many scholars have noted that HIV-related illness saps sexual desire and energy (e.g., Hoffman, 1991), but few have given attention to the pragmatic challenges faced by those individuals who remain healthy and sexually active.

Finally, two women, one with a 10-year-old son, commented on the lack of attention to the unique experiences of women who are living with HIV and AIDS. They noted, for example, that HIV-positive women will enter menopause in their 20s and 30s with no psychological preparation for this transition. They noted that support groups are composed primarily of gay men whose concerns are quite different from theirs. In fact, one of these women started the first support group for women in the city of Chicago. "It was hard," she said, "to find other women like me, who were experiencing what I was experiencing, but I knew that I had to if I was going to survive." She also described the problems of parenting when one is HIV positive and one's child is HIV negative. She commented that "when my husband became severely debilitated, he started to push our son away cause he didn't want him to get hurt when he died . . . but he was okay with it; he always knew it would happen. He's okay with me too. We focus on quality, not quantity of time." Then she added, "I have already had my son adopted by one of my friends. My family doesn't want him—or me. Now that's something you should study: Who takes care of the children when mom in gone?"

CONCLUSION

We have presented here the experiences of people who go about the business of living despite the fact that they are HIV positive or have AIDS. Many have lost their jobs, their friends, and their health, but most have not lost their spirit. They volunteered to share their experiences because they wanted others to understand their problems, their resourcefulness, their commonness, and their diversity. We hope that we have presented their stories as they would want them told.

RELEVANT CONCEPTS

coping strategies
emotion-regulating coping
problem-solving coping
rejection
relational consequences
resignation with purpose
social support

DISCUSSION QUESTIONS

1. Why is AIDS considered a "stigmatized" disease and how does this stigma disenfranchise persons who are HIV positive or who have AIDS (PWAs)?

2. What are relevant issues of social support from friends, family, and acquaintances of persons who are HIV positive or have AIDS? Why might some potential supporters pull away whereas others offer sustained support?

3. Discuss the media's coverage of AIDS and its impact on society's attitudes and behaviors toward persons who are HIV positive or have AIDS.

4. In what ways, if any, have persons who are HIV positive or have AIDS become enfranchised?

5. Do we have an obligation to identify persons who are HIV positive or have AIDS and make that knowledge known to previous partners, employers, and so forth? Why or why not?

SUGGESTED READINGS

Callen, M. (1990). *Surviving AIDS.* New York: HarperCollins.

Cherry, K., & Smith, D. (1993). Sometimes I cry: The experience of loneliness for men with AIDS. *Health Communication, 5*, 181–208.

Hoffman, M. A. (1991). Counseling the HIV-infected client: A psychological assessment and intervention. *The Counseling Psychologist, 19*, 467–542.

Lazarus, R., & Folkman, S. (1984). *Stress, appraisal, and coping.* New York: Springer.

Namir, S., Alumbaught, M. M., Fawzy, F. I., & Wolcott, D. L. (1989). The relationship of support to physical aspects of AIDS. *Psychology and Health, 3*, 77–86.

Weitz, R. (1990). Living with the stigma of AIDS. *Qualitative Sociology, 13*, 23–28.

15 "Stripping You of Everything You Ever Held Dear to Your Heart": The Many Losses of Women With HIV/AIDS

Rebecca J. Welch Cline
University of Florida

Nelya J. McKenzie
Auburn University at Montgomery

AIDS is a stigmatizing disease and a disease of the already stigmatized. In the United States, the social construction of AIDS cast it as a gay man's disease. The resulting failure to associate women with HIV/AIDS rendered them invisible in the epidemic. Society at large has failed to identify women with HIV/AIDS to a large degree because women were virtually ignored in the scientific and educational literature for the first decade of the epidemic (Cline & McKenzie, 1996b). The resulting inattention has only added to the burden of women with the disease.

People who are stigmatized are treated as the outcasts of society in their personal relationships and in their social encounters at large. The tendency to identify AIDS only with gay men adds "homosexual" to the aspersions cast on women with AIDS. Women with AIDS tend to be associated, naively, with prostitution and promiscuity and are judged particularly harshly due to a double standard of sexuality. Further, the epidemiology of women with AIDS in the United States clearly identifies additional stigma for women with AIDS: Women with AIDS tend to be women of color, women coping with poverty, women alone caring for children, and women already challenged to receive quality health care. Numerous threads of stigma lead to the disenfranchisement of women with HIV/AIDS, who suffer additional losses unique to their gender in the context of HIV disease (Cline & McKenzie, 1996a).

STIGMA, WOMEN, AND HIV/AIDS

In practice, stigma divides the world into "us" and "them." The identification of a discrediting attribute functions to undermine one group while labeling another "normal" or desirable (Goffman, 1963). People with AIDS, regardless of gender or mode of transmission, are stigmatized by the meanings associated with the disease. Both men and women with AIDS suffer from multiple stigmatizing associations: homosexuality, IV drug use, the stigma of dying. Ironically an HIV diagnosis enhances one's need for social support at the same time that the label tends to undermine one's interpersonal relationships. The result is distancing, if not abandonment, rejection, and judgment. Research indicates that both family members and friends (McDonell, Abell, & Miller, 1991), as well as health professionals (Kelly, St. Lawrence, Smith, Hood, & Cook, 1987), typically respond to persons with AIDS (PWAs) with sufficient rejection as to withhold social support and adequate physical and medical care. The typical PWA feels anxious, depressed, alienated, distressed, and estranged from others. However, the degree of ostracism *felt* is related directly to *how* stigmatized one feels (Crandall & Coleman, 1992), and generally women feel more stigmatized by AIDS than do their gay male counterparts.

Beyond the "typical" rejection experienced by PWAs, women with HIV/AIDS *experience* even greater stigmatization, in part because they do not *expect* to be stigmatized (Crandall & Coleman, 1992). Moreover, women's gender socialization adds to their disenfranchisement in the contexts of prevention and living with an HIV diagnosis. Because women tend to be defined "in relation to" others, the disease threatens not only their health but their very identities. For example, many women who may wish to practice safer sex find themselves powerless to do so in the context of gender roles that demand compliance with their partners' demands; some fear physical abuse as well as relational loss in this context (e.g., Richardson, 1990). Women who contract HIV are judged harshly by a sexual double standard, relative to their male heterosexual counterparts, as being "easy" or "promiscuous." The result is that women tend to be blamed disportionately for spreading the disease (e.g., the overemphasis on prostitution relative to its nearly nonexistent role in the epidemic in the United States) both to men and to their children.

Beyond the blame of others, women with HIV/AIDS often blame themselves for their role losses as mother and provider. The role of mother is critical to the self-worth of many women who live on the margins of society due to race or poverty. The pregnant HIV-infected woman, faced with a decision to terminate pregnancy or not, encounters the potential loss of her role as mother versus the possibility that she may not live to provide for the child that may well be healthy. Women with HIV/AIDS are disproportionately poor and often are the key, if not only, caregivers for other family members. The result is that they are likely to expend their energy and resources on others while neglecting their own health needs. Thus, the potential losses for women of their roles as partner, mother, and care provider threaten women with HIV/AIDS and often interfere with their own health and social care.

Women with AIDS often are minorities who are coping with poverty, large families, low education, and limited social support. Many do not have knowledge of, or access to, the basic health, social, and legal services they need to cope with their situations. Their initial risk to the disease, and their later lack of ability to cope with it, shrink in meaning in the context of "homelessness, joblessness, starvation, and abandonment" (Nyamathi & Vasquez, 1989, p. 300). Thus, the everyday challenge for many women with HIV/AIDS is survival.

This chapter focuses on two women, Donna and Linda. They have responded to having HIV/AIDS by being very public with their condition as they participate actively in AIDS education and prevention efforts. However, they face certain dilemmas that are particularly salient to women with the disease.

BACKGROUND

Although Donna and Linda differ in age, lifestyle, and mode of transmission of the HIV virus, their initial and subsequent experiences relative to being diagnosed HIV positive were similar.

Donna

Donna is 35 years old, has a high school education, and is unemployed. Her most recent employment was as a seamstress at a factory that produces seats for vans. She is attractive, articulate, and intelligent. In addition, Donna is readily likable. She is the prototype of a person "who doesn't look like she has AIDS." Nevertheless, Donna does have AIDS. Her income is limited to disability benefits from Social Security (SSI) and what she earns as a speaker for the local AIDS network. She is married and has no children. Although Donna has a history of cocaine use, which resulted in a prison sentence, she has been "clean" for many years. She found out she was HIV positive in 1985 after donating blood:

> I was in a bad car accident in 1981 and just about lost my life. I made it through in part due to a blood transfusion that I received. So when I came out of that I decided I needed to pay back whoever it was that had saved

> my life. So, for years I donated blood. And not until they started testing blood did I find out. I got a letter in the mail—a registered letter saying come to the blood bank. And I couldn't even go at the time I got the letter. They set me up an appointment like a week or so later. Immediately, there was only one thing that I could think, because it was right after they first started testing blood for it [HIV/AIDS].

Donna indicated that structured social support was not important to her in the early days of her diagnosis: "I didn't feel I had a need for it at the time." However, after being prescribed AZT she sought a support group: "When I got put on AZT, that's when I needed the support. Because, I couldn't believe it. It was like getting told all over again that I was sick. I felt I was too healthy. I couldn't believe that I was going to have to go on AZT. And, I kinda fell apart over that. So I started going to a support group." Since that time, Donna has been committed to both giving and receiving social support through the local AIDS network.

Linda

Linda is 27 years old, has a high school education and about 2 years of postsecondary education. She has a 9-year-old daughter who lives with the child's father. Linda also has AIDS and is unemployed. Her most recent employment was as a secretary at a local hospital. Like Donna, Linda's income consists of SSI and what she earns speaking for the local AIDS network. She is fairly attractive and extremely open about her AIDS status and history of IV drug use (IVDU) and prostitution. Despite her IVDU and prostitution status, it was a "bad car deal" that sent her to prison for over a year. Shortly after her release from prison, Linda found out that she was HIV positive:

> They had me tested in prison. Of course 99% of the people they tested in prison were positive because the testing they did was not accurate. They told me I was on a list of being exposed. They ran one test and it came up positive. They ran another one and lost it. Then I got released. When I came to University City in March of 1990, I started testing then and my test came out positive, HIV positive. But, I don't know if I got it [HIV virus] from needles or from sex.

Linda's attitude about a "structured" support system differs drastically from that of Donna. Linda does not go to a support group, explaining: "I don't want to go somewhere where I hear everybody talk about how they're feeling, what their pains are, because I already know. I like to be out there in society where people are feeling great, having a good time, 'cause that's me. They [the health department] suggested to me to join a support group, but I just—support groups aren't something I'm really into." Rather than a structured support group, Linda indicated that individuals can be supportive of her if they followed the advice: "Be yourself. I don't want you to be anything other than yourself when you're around me. I don't ask anybody for anything except if I need to speak to you, just give me that time."

Both of these women strive to live a life of normalcy in the face of often seemingly insurmountable obstacles. As AIDS educators, they demonstrate an exceptional willingness to share their stories, serving as constant reminders of the urgent need for AIDS education and prevention. However, other less noticeable aspects of their lives serve to remind us of the enormous courage women with AIDS must display in the day-to-day course of living with AIDS. Both of these women have experienced the effects of stigma (including the association of AIDS with homosexuality), the loss of traditional gender roles (particularly that of being a mother), difficulty in obtaining health care targeted to women with HIV/AIDS, and affronts to their dignity induced by the heavy financial burden of living with HIV/AIDS.

STIGMA AND INTERPERSONAL RELATIONS

Both Donna and Linda disclosed their HIV status almost immediately to their closest friends and family. Although neither of the women experienced rejection by those closest to them, the disclosure resulted in some unexpected reactions from the people with whom they were closest.

Donna

Even before Donna received official notice of her HIV status, she revealed her suspicions to one of her roommates. After receiving a registered letter from the blood bank where she had been a recent donor, Donna told her roommate, "I know that it's AIDS." However, her fears seemed groundless. "I didn't have any kind of symptoms or anything. Didn't know anybody [with AIDS]. I had no sexual partners that were sick from AIDS or anything like that in my past. It's just that inside sunk feeling."

Despite a promise of confidentiality, the roommate told Donna's other roommate about the test results. Donna says that after learning about the betrayal, "I made it very obvious that I had another blood test appointment and I came back and told them the test came back negative. Nothing was wrong and it was all a mistake. And for a long time they believed that." In truth, however, "All the blood tests came back obviously the same":

> It really hurt my feelings bad. Because here I not only went through such a devastation, but I was betrayed by my best friend. I understand now that it was a hard thing to lay on her and expect to keep to herself. But we went through a period of separation over it. Because when something like that comes along and you feel you need to confide in somebody, you need that privacy. You need that confidante to be exactly that, somebody that you can talk to and trust. And if I would have said it did not matter, like now it doesn't matter who knows, that would be different. But at that time it was not a big social issue of acceptance. People did not accept it then. It was something new to everybody. It was only gays and drug users that got it. And even today people still want to insist that you must have been an IV drug user or you must have been out whoring around. They still don't want to accept that normal people can get it.

As one would expect, Donna was unsure about in whom to confide about her HIV status. "I did not want anybody to know because I knew how I had thought [about people with AIDS] and I didn't want people to think that way about me. I didn't want the stigma that went along with it." One obvious choice was her fiancé, whose reaction frightened rather than comforted her: "He kinda scared me more about it by telling me not to tell anybody. And he told me after I told my roommate that I shouldn't have done that. He was right, for the hurt that it caused me, but he made me more afraid of anybody finding out by the way he was talking about it. I guess I hadn't thought about it the same way that he had. In that fearful kind of way."

Donna described her parents as being very supportive. However, deeply entrenched myths about how the HIV virus is spread led to some initial hurtful reactions:

> My mom and dad both were very positive. The whole family is. Then when I went home for my brother's wedding and I was staying at my mom's house, I'd get up in the morning and I'd drink my cup of coffee. And all the dirty dishes would go on one side of the sink. And my mom would take my coffee cup and she would put it over on the other side of the sink and say, "Don't put your dishes over here with everybody else's." It hurt. It really hurt, bad. And I told her, "Mom, you can't get it that way." And she says "Well, I'm not worried about me. I'm worried about your grandmother." But I know that she wasn't just worried about my grandmother.

Linda

Linda indicated that, with the exception of her daughter, "I don't have any family." After learning of her HIV status, Linda told her child's father. "Since I told him, he's gotten her tested and himself and they're both negative. I was relieved, real relieved."

In describing her feelings about her past association with others, Linda admits to feelings of guilt. She indicated that, "At first the guilt that I felt was overwhelming. To think, oh shit, whose life did I ruin." She was able to get past the guilt "because I have notified everybody myself and who I couldn't notify myself the health department did. And it's a relief when you make that step." However, she feels especially responsible for her partner of 5 years:

> Guilt—having to tell my partner of 5 years that I was infected and that I may have infected him. But he will not test. He doesn't want to know. I have tried to get him to test. I have begged; I have pleaded. I have sent the health department. He doesn't want to know. He stays in denial as far as I'm concerned. He doesn't want to believe that I have AIDS. He feels like there's a big miracle happening somewhere and overnight I'm going to be cured. I think he has some guilt hanging over him because he has been promiscuous while he was with me. He started naming all these names. I feel that he should notify the people, but I don't know if he's done that or if he will.

Linda indicated that her partner of 5 years was the first person she told when she found out she was HIV positive. Although she has become very open about her condition, his response has been to avoid public disclosure:

> He wants me to shelter myself, to shut myself away from people. He's not comfortable with my openness. I think it's the social aspect. You know, what people are going to think about him and him being with someone with AIDS. Whether they know that he has contracted it or not really doesn't matter. It's just the fact that he's with someone with AIDS. And it's an ego thing, really. His mother is a minister and I guess he's afraid that if certain people find out he'll be crushed. But I told his mother and to me she's fine. But he tells me that she doesn't want him to come over to her house and do laundry anymore because of my AIDS. I haven't seen that, so I don't believe what he's saying. I just think it's in his mind.

Despite her partner's attempts to keep her "shut away," Linda continues to be very open about her AIDS status. "I come right out and say, I have AIDS. I don't hide it; I'm not ashamed of it. I'm here to educate." During her "openness," Linda has had only two negative reactions to her HIV status:

> Now people are learning more about it, you know. They hear about it and read about it and most everyone I come in contact with knows how they can contract the virus. So, I have encountered only two people that have really backed away. One was a guy tripping on acid and he kinda freaked out. And one was a girl that I used to go to school with. I saw her in the

> grocery store one night and she said, "I heard," and all of a sudden she backed up 20 feet. Chalk it up to ignorance.

Even though, as Linda indicated, people know more about HIV/AIDS today than in the early days of the epidemic, people, as Donna stated, "still don't want to accept that normal people can get it." Part of the perception of "normal" people includes heterosexuality. These women found their sexuality was at times suspect because of their HIV status.

HOMOSEXUAL?

Donna

Although uncommon, Donna reported that the question of her sexual preference has been raised, supporting the stereotype that people with AIDS are homosexual:

> The question's been raised because I was in jail for a period of time. And so, the people that I worked with at my last job—the women that I worked with—I talked to one of the women on the phone one time and she says, "Well, everybody up at work said that you got it while you were in prison." And I said, "Excuse me?" And it didn't dawn on me at the time. It just made me mad. I said, "No, I didn't get it there." And then when I told my husband, he says, "Well, what are they saying? That you're gay?" And that's when it dawned on me. That's what I mean about people trying to say that it can't happen to a normal person.

Linda

Linda reported less concern with questions about her sexuality. As she stated:

> I have people ask me if I'm heterosexual or bisexual. And they want to know that, I guess, to see if they're at risk. I guess if they are homosexual—female—to see if they're at risk to contract the virus. The male homosexual myth, you know. But, I haven't really encountered much of that. You know, people ask me, but I don't hide anything.

Despite the threats to their interpersonal relationships and questions about their sexuality that stem from the stigma associated with HIV/AIDS, both women indicated that the loss of their identity as a mother is the most tragic aspect of the disease.

ROLE LOSSES

Guidelines from the Centers for Disease Control (CDC) recommend that women with HIV/AIDS forego pregnancy. The implication of such a recommendation is serious for these women. Specifically, bearing a child often is seen as "an irresponsible and selfish act if the woman is HIV infected" (Anastos & Marte, 1989, p. 10). However, the probability of HIV transmission from mother to fetus has been estimated to be as low as 20% (Stratton, Mofenson, & Willoughby, 1992). Nevertheless, the CDC "guideline" often translates into a "directive," as women with AIDS give up one of their most defining characteristics, that of mother.

Donna

For Donna, who has no children, the decision to remain childless has been painful:

> When we became involved, I told him [husband], "You know, we've got to think about a lot of things." For me the hardest thing with the disease, and even now sometimes it's difficult for me, is not being able to have children. Because that's the one thing that I always wanted. When I got married I wanted to have my own home, have my own children. And I felt that I had gone through all my heyday of drinking and partying and snorting cocaine. I went to jail. I cleaned myself up and straightened my whole life out. I was involved in a church and doing all the right things and then all of a sudden I get this letter in the mail and I get slapped in the face with, well, it doesn't do you any good to straighten out now. And so the hardest thing for me was to be able to talk about not having children. And up until about a year or so ago I couldn't even say it. I would just totally break down.

In an almost desperate desire to be a mother, Donna sought alternative parenting arrangements:

> I even went so far as to try to become a foster parent. I was thinking, well, I could become a foster parent to AIDS babies or something like that. I was just grasping at straws. Being a foster parent is not a practical thing to do because I can't be around the children when they are sick. If they became infected with something, that might infect me. I can't be around them. And something else I found out is that people who have any kind of terminal illness are not allowed to adopt children. So, it's a hurtful thing all the way around. And that has probably been the most devastating part of this disease for me.

As with most young married women of child-bearing age, others also expected Donna to have children. Ironically, treatment for the very disease that precluded pregnancy led those Donna worked with to think she actually was pregnant:

> When I had to go on the AZT they put me on ten pills a day. And AZT is a very, very strong drug. I was sick all the time. The people I was working with, I couldn't tell them what I had. Nobody knew. My family was all that knew. And people knew how much I loved children and that I always wanted to have children. So the women that I used to work with would kid me all the time because I was constantly throwing up. I mean I was in and out of the bathroom. I was always sick. And they were always kidding me, "Oh, you must be pregnant." Little did they know that I—that was absolutely impossible.

Not only did Donna experience the loss of "mother role" for herself, but she also felt an extended loss for her mother who now would not become a grandmother. As Donna explained, "She was upset that I was sick and upset at the fact that there go all chances of me having any grandchildren for her."

Linda

Unlike Donna, Linda has a child, although the child does not live with her. As a young woman, Linda had anticipated having another child at some point in time. However, the anticipation of having a second child ended when she tested positive for the HIV virus:

> I explain to them [audiences] first and foremost I am a mother. I get a little frustrated about knowing that I can't have any more children. Well, let me say it like this. It's not that I can't, it's that I won't because I'm infected and there's a 50% [estimates often are lower than 50%] chance that the child is going to be infected. Why do I want to give birth to a child who I know is only going to live to be either 2 or, at the very most, 6 years old? That's probably the hardest thing for me to deal with. I've dealt with the death and the dying and everything else. Now, I also have to deal with the fact that I have only one child and there won't be any more.

As a result of gynecological problems associated with AIDS, Linda is scheduled for a hysterectomy, eliminating *any* possibility of her having another child. A friend of Linda's who also is HIV positive, described Linda's situation in a way that demonstrates the unique capacity of women to provide social support for other women relative to this particular female loss:

> I went over to see Linda. She was all upset. And it can make you feel better when you can talk to another person. I've already had a hysterectomy in my life, so I can tell her something about it. But she's so young. She was really upset because of having to have a hysterectomy. Not that she should even have another baby. It was just the idea, mentally for her.

Although the loss of their role as mother may be the most emotionally devastating aspect of HIV/AIDS for these women, other losses are experienced as they seek ways to acquire medical care appropriate for women with AIDS.

QUALITY OF HEALTH CARE

The typical woman with AIDS is poor. People with AIDS, in general, are challenged to find and afford quality health care. Many health care providers hold the same negative stereotypes and reflect the same prejudices of PWAs as the general public; as a result, many are reluctant to treat PWAs. The health care system particularly challenges women with HIV and in some unique ways. Because women do not fit the stereotype of a person with AIDS held by health care providers, often they are not diagnosed early and sometimes have difficulty seeing themselves as a candidate for HIV infection and for AIDS as the disease progresses. In turn, they may not seek health care quickly and when they do, often they have particular difficulty finding adequate care.

Donna

Donna's reaction to testing positive is a common one—denial, a response that initially kept her from seeking health care and social support:

> I totally did not believe it first when I found out. I think I went partying almost every night for like weeks and weeks and weeks because I just couldn't believe that could happen to me. But I did go for three different blood tests within the next eight months. 'Cause I was sure they made a mistake. It could not have happened. And all the blood tests came back obviously the same. [I thought] it was only gays and drug users that got it, you know . . . people still don't accept that normal people can get it.

Like many women diagnosed with HIV, Donna's denial prevented her from seeking treatment immediately: "When I first found out, I never ever took any medications and I ignored it and I never got any treatment or even found out anything. . . . just ignored it. 'Cause I didn't know what else to do."

Donna's residence, when she was diagnosed with HIV, was in Central County; however, she found that she could not get adequate care in that rural area:

> When I originally moved to Central City, I called the 1-800-FLA-AIDS [information line] and got connected with a so-called doctor down in Central City, who advised me at the time, which has been now almost 4 years ago, not to seek services or help in that county. They said "You will not find a doctor in Central County to treat you." They recommended that I go to North County for help. And they were right. Because we went through the whole phone book of doctors and only five said, "Oh, yeah, we can take you." But when we'd call back they'd say, "Oh, well, I'm sorry but . . . we can't take any new patients."

Thus, Donna's search for health care confirmed what she was told; she was forced to go outside of her county to receive care. She soon found herself referring others to North County for the same reasons: "I refer so many people up here . . . for the hospital services. Like for dental. We don't have anybody to cover dental down there. One dentist does normal cleanings, but nobody in Central City is ready to take on that responsibility." Donna's experiences in Central City soon educated her about the need for, and the absence of, care by doctors specifically knowledgeable about AIDS:

> The state health department had not had a doctor in there who is AIDS aware. I mean they've got a doctor in there who is more of a pediatric doctor taking care of AIDS patients . . . if he were trained he could be capable, but he's not. And he does the best he can with it but you can't just go in and say "Okay I know this doctor knows what he is doing and I feel safe." I know better because he almost killed me. They're not infectious disease specialists. He's just a doctor who goes by basic guidelines of being careful with certain diseases . . . but he doesn't know how to treat PWAs or the results of some of their medications.

Donna pointed out that the lack of quality gynecological services was a health care need specific to women with AIDS in her area: "If they could find somebody to refer us to other than the health department all the time. The health department will do it but if you have some heavy-duty female problems, [they aren't good]. I just wish they could find a gynecologist who would take HIV-infected people and not have any qualms about it."

When Donna began to rely on the local AIDS network in North County she ran into bureaucratic barriers because she was receiving treatment in a locale other than where she lived: "They found out up here . . . that I was getting involved in the support group up here . . . and then somebody that I was having a disagreement with in Central City called up here and turned me in for the fact that I was going out of the county for treatment." Donna's husband, Joe, described what happened as a result:

> They cut her off from her treatment up here and sent her to Central County and they almost killed her down there. She became very sick. Okay, they used the wrong drugs; they changed her whole treatment program. From place to place, the doctors, the quality of care is very important. And they almost killed her. And that's when I said, "That's it! Keep your mouth shut from now on. . . . We'll get you some care." And that's what we did.

Linda

Linda was concerned about her HIV status both because of where she lives and because of her own behavioral risks. She said, "It was always on my mind everyday." So, in 1989, she began to get tested: "My background is 6 years of IV drug use. After stopping that I went fully into prostitution and I've been clean for 5 years. But it was always on my mind . . . Beach County has a high infection rate. So I'd been testing since November of '89. But every fifth test was coming up positive and they weren't going by Florida statutes and doing follow-up tests . . ." Although she only recently has been diagnosed with AIDS in North County, she believes she was positive much earlier and that faulty testing failed to identify her status accurately. In fact, because no follow-up tests were being done, she kept going back for more tests on her own. At the same time, regardless of her test result each time, no counseling was provided to her, either about the meaning of the test or how she could prevent infection: "They just told you and let you deal with it." When she finally was tested in North County and got her results, like Donna, Linda responded with denial: "I just didn't believe it. I did and I didn't. I kept saying 'No this isn't right.' I kept saying 'Something's wrong, you know. They're not doing something right.' " At the same time she felt some relief because she finally had an answer to explain her numerous health problems, an answer that her doctors apparently had failed to consider: "I was relieved when they told me I was HIV positive because I knew what was wrong with my body now. I just kept having things that were going wrong and I couldn't get any answers."

At present, Linda feels like she is getting more than adequate health care. She is part of a program called "We Care" that locates health care providers who specialize in the field needed. "As far as health care in general for the virus, I get excellent health care." Her primary health care is provided by the health department and paid for by Medicaid; she qualifies because she has no income. Although she characterizes her care as "excellent," she acknowledges that her inability to provide her own health insurance prevents her from getting the kind of care she would prefer: "I would like to be back working in a place of business where I have insurance, where I could get things done faster, you now, such as surgery." Linda also identified the need for more and better gynecological care as a specific need for herself and for other women with HIV/AIDS in her area. She noted that the many gynecological manifestations of the disease magnify the need for gynecological care by someone with HIV specialization.

FINANCIAL BURDEN

Unfortunately, the quality of health care received corresponds directly to one's ability to pay. However, the financial burden of getting adequate health care is only one of many financial challenges faced by women with AIDS. This theme reverberates through both Linda's and Donna's portrayals of their everyday experiences of coping with HIV/AIDS.

Donna

Like Linda, Donna is unemployed and has been forced to rely on "the system" for assistance to help her manage the financial crisis created by her disease:

> Nobody expects that this early in life that this kind of thing is going to happen. You don't have anything set away as a savings. And you have nothing to fall back on when you want to be a normal person. You still want normal things. You still need new shoes. You still need to be able to feel that once in awhile you can go buy a new dress . . . and look nice and decent. . . . And to be totally zapped out of any kind of financial capacity . . . I live on less [for a month] than most people make in a week. And that is hard to do. And there's a demeaning aspect of it. I'm limited and most times I can't even get the bills down.

Donna's husband, Joe, describes being forced to provide misinformation to the bureaucracy about dates and locations of treatment in order to ensure Donna gets adequate care. Her situation was exacerbated further in Central City when the health department decided that she had the financial resources to support her own AZT treatments:

> They said, "Oh, we understand you own a home and you have this and you have that and you have lots of jewelry and you have grands and grands of money in the bank." And I'm like thinking they are crazy. They said "Can I see a paystub?" I said, "Excuse me, I'm unemployed. I don't know where

you're getting your information from but. . . ." They said, "I want to see a paystub from you and him [her husband] both." Neither of us were employed, you know. Yeah, we have a home but there's no equity in it. We just bought it 'cause the guy was practically giving it away. And we borrowed the money to get in it, . . . a minimal down payment. And we had to do it then because we knew when my HIV got worse you can't get the loan. So we did it. Now, for sure I wouldn't be able to get a home.

Not only the bureaucracy, but society as a whole adds to the financial burden by stigmatizing PWAs when they cannot pay for their care. Donna explained that the financial burden is bad enough without others' judgments:

> My diamond ring here, people look at that and they think "How can you possibly need help wearing a rock like that?" You know, people will comment on it. Well, I had this before any of this happened. I mean, this is my wedding ring! What am I supposed to do? Hock everything that I own and give up—they kind of force you into giving up all of your dignity and anything you ever worked for in your life. You're just supposed to give it up. And that's not how it should be. I mean, it's bad enough to have to deal with this disease, let alone stripping you of everything that you've every held hear to your heart and worked for.

One of Donna's many financial challenges is paying for health insurance. Medicaid is her only other alternative and to qualify for Medicaid:

> They said I had to be divorced from my husband, could not being living with him and had to be destitute. Destitute! I said "Fine. I'm packing my bag. He'll drop me off at your front step at Medicaid Administration . . . and then you can find me a place to eat, to live. Figure out a way that I am going to eat. Figure out who's going to pay medical bills. And then you can tell me how destitute I am." Oh, they about had a fit. "Don't do that Mrs. Gallagher, it's okay." I said, "Well don't you tell me that . . . I'll become destitute real fast."

Donna described the assistance she has gotten from the local AIDS network for covering the cost of her health insurance: "For me, my insurance premiums I haven't been able to pay. And our network down there [Central City] won't pay for it or wouldn't at the time. Because I am a client up here and in the speaker's bureau and support groups and stuff, they said 'Okay, we'll put it to a vote.' " The local network covered Donna's premiums of nearly $150 a month for 3 months: "They know that we don't want people to have to go on Medicaid. You know that's your last resort. And you obviously get better treatment when you have more money."

A tone of desperation came through as Joe described the efforts he and Donna have made to try to keep her health insurance:

> I'm going to drop mine . . . I can't keep up with it this month. But hers, I had to put it on credit cards. . . . I can't let it lapse. I've sold jewelry. I've sold anything I can sell. I've turned in stocks, bonds, things that I had from the past. I've done everything I could and now I'm down to where there is nothing else to get rid of but personal things. And that's going to hurt people emotionally if that starts happening. . . . And you look around and say, "Where am I going to turn? Where can I go for help? Who can understand?"

Donna explained that her eligibility for special support in order to finance her health care has run out and that now she must prove she is disabled in order to get assistance. However, in turn, her insurance premiums went up: "Then the premiums go up to 150% and that's like 170-something for my premiums, which is ridiculous. When you're disabled you can't pay for anything anyway. And then they do it [raise the premiums] . . . to try to discourage you and to drop you [from coverage]. They want to get rid of you and those AZT bills."

Donna's treatment alone costs an average of $800 per month. Unfortunately, the cost of health care and health insurance are only a part of the financial challenge faced by women with AIDS:

> One of the biggest parts of it, besides keeping a positive mental attitude is your nutrition. You have to eat right. Have to eat fresh vegetables and lean meats and you have to constantly eat, even when you don't feel like it. You have to. And in order to do that it costs money. I mean, just for Joe and myself, in order for me to eat properly it's close to $100 a week that I'm going to have to spend in groceries. Well, I'm not doing that right now because I don't have it.

Linda

Linda is unemployed; she has no income, depends on food stamps for food, and relies heavily on the assistance she receives from the local AIDS network for meeting her housing needs. Although she has become adept at making "the system" work for her, lack of financial resources for basic survival needs is a constant concern. Linda gets some help from the local AIDS network for participating in the speaker's bureau but even an organization whose mission is to facilitate care for PWAs seems insensitive, in Linda's eyes, to her financial realities:

> I am always fighting to get my money from speaking engagements and it shouldn't be that way. It might be 2 or 3 weeks before I got paid. Plus speaking engagements are supposed to be distributed on a rotation basis but they aren't. And it takes too long to get your money. They don't seem to understand the need to get the money immediately. They don't understand

how important $25 is to somebody. I'm not able to work and $25 is important to me. And I need it right away.

Although most of her health care is provided by Medicaid, she has to pay for some of her drugs. She relies heavily on friends at a distance for social support and said that managing her phone bill is difficult.

Linda may survive the financial challenges better than many women because she is "street wise" to "the system." She is well aware of the degree of her dependency on Medicaid, the health department, and the AIDS network. She readily admitted that "there's a way to beat the system" that otherwise requires a person to liquidate her assets in order to get meaningful assistance. For Linda this means planning interactions with representatives of the bureaucracy and being practiced at looking "destitute": "When I go into Social Security I look like I'm dying. I don't put any makeup on, don't take any medications. I don't take any pain pills. I've lost a lot of weight and so I just go in there and I wear bicycle shorts, something that really shows how small you are." Like many women with HIV/AIDS, Linda feels forced to misrepresent her situation in order to survive:

I give them one address but I live in another. My fiancé says that I live there and that he's taking care of me to the best of his ability, but in reality I live in another home by myself, take care of myself . . . and I don't have a vehicle but you can't put a vehicle in your name. You have to put them in a friend's name, someone you can trust. And I've been burned . . . on four vehicles . . . Ralph [the person she trusted] still got 'em all.

A TAPESTRY OF LOSSES

Woven together, the various threads of stigma for women with HIV/AIDS yield a tapestry of disenfranchisement in which interpersonal relationships become intensely challenging, if not the source of rejection. One's social worth is threatened by stereotypes associated with the disease. One's identity as a woman is threatened at the prospect of significant role losses. One's health and well-being are threatened not only by the disease but by prejudice in a health care system that fails to identify women with the disease. And one's survival is threatened by the sheer absence of financial and social resources requisite to sustaining everyday life.

RELEVANT CONCEPTS

denial
gender role

identity management
interpersonal relationships
role loss
self-concept
self-disclosure
social support
stigma

DISCUSSION QUESTIONS

1. Compare and contrast how women with HIV/AIDS and men with HIV/AIDS are stigmatized in their interpersonal relationships and by society at large. In what ways are the dilemmas they face similar? In what ways are they different?

2. Women with HIV/AIDS face the dilemma of disclosing their physical condition to others in their personal and professional lives and in their interactions with "the system." Weigh the risks and benefits of total honesty in these disclosures as evidenced by Linda and Donna. Using their experiences as a starting point, consider the impact of making or withholding those disclosures on whether the women receive optimal instrumental and emotional social support.

3. Symbolic interactionist theorists contend that, to a large degree, the self is defined through interactions with others, specifically via the various roles that we play. From this perspective, what are the challenges faced by Donna and Linda, in particular, and by women with HIV/AIDS, in general, in terms of maintaining strong self-concepts?

4. Although Donna and Linda reported different attitudes about reliance on social support groups per se, in what ways do their accounts indicate a *need* for social support? How did the two women go about assuring that their needs for social support were met? How might their needs for social support differ from those of men with HIV/AIDS?

5. Numerous public and private organizations exist, in part, to provide social support to people with AIDS. These include community networks, county and state health departments, insurance programs, and health care organizations. Assume that you have been hired as a consultant by one of these organizations to advise them on how to most efficiently and effectively serve their clientele. You have specific and well-founded evidence that the PWAs attempting to access support via this organization often find themselves being "stripped" of "everything you ever held dear to your heart." Imagine that you are going to do a briefing for management. Include the following: (a) an explanation of the "nature of the problem," that is, what

the "problem" is as experienced by PWAs, and (b) a set of guidelines for the organization to facilitate their interpersonal and bureaucratic interactions with PWAs.

REFERENCES/SUGGESTED READINGS

Anastos, K., & Marte, C. (1989). Women: The missing persons in the AIDS epidemic. *Health/PAC Bulletin, 19*(4), 6–13.

Cline, R. J. W., & McKenzie, N. J. (1996a). HIV/AIDS, women, and threads of discrimination: A tapestry of disenfranchisement. In E. B. Ray (Ed.), *Communication and disenfranchisement: Social health issues and implications*. Mahwah, NJ: Lawrence Erlbaum Associates.

Cline, R. J. W., & McKenzie, N. J. (1996b). Women and AIDS: The lost population. In R. L. Parrott & C. M. Condit (Eds.), *Evaluating women's health messages: A resource book* (pp. 382–401). Newbury Park, CA: Sage.

Crandall, C. S., & Coleman, R. (1992). AIDS-related stigmatization and the disruption of social relationships. *Journal of Social and Personal Relationships, 9*, 163–177.

Goffman, E. (1963). *Stigma: Notes on the management of spoiled identity*. Englewood Cliffs, NJ: Prentice-Hall.

Kelly, J. A., St. Lawrence, J. S., Smith, S., Hood, H. V., & Cook, D. J. (1987). Stigmatization of AIDS patients by physicians. *American Journal of Public Health, 77*, 789–791.

McDonell, N. R., Abell, N., & Miller, J. (1991). Family members' willingness to care for people with AIDS: A psychosocial assessment model. *Social Work, 36*, 43–53.

Nyamathi, A., & Vasquez, R. (1989). Impact of poverty, homelessness, and drugs on Hispanic women at risk for HIV infection. *Hispanic Journal of Behavioral Sciences, 11*, 299–314.

Richardson, D. (1990). AIDS education and women: Sexual and reproductive issues. In P. Aggleton, P. Davies, & G. Hart (Eds.), *AIDS: Individual, cultural, and policy dimensions* (pp. 169–179). London: Palmer Press.

Stratton, P., Mofenson, L., & Willoughby, A. (1992). Human immunodeficiency virus infection in pregnant women under care at AIDS clinical trial centers in the United States. *Obstetrics & Gynecology, 79*, 364–368.

16 *"But I Don't Know What to Say to Her": Communication With the Terminally Ill*

Teresa L. Thompson
University of Dayton

Kim Schmidt put down her spade and rubbed her shoulder once again. She must be getting old, she thought. Although 44 didn't seem old to her mind, her body was feeling the years. Her shoulder, in particular, seemed to hurt all the time anymore. She was never going to get any gardening done the way it was feeling. She had planned on getting all the impatiens planted before her youngest kids got home from school, but reluctantly decided that the rest of the flowers would have to wait until tomorrow.

Turning, she heard a shouted, "Kim!" from the street. Her two closest friends, Kelley and Sara, waved her toward them. They were evidently returning from one of their daily walks, part of their attempt to turn to a more healthy lifestyle. Still rubbing her shoulder and grimacing, Kim walked toward them.

"Is your shoulder hurting you again?" asked Kelley with concern. "I told you to see Steve about that." Kelley's husband, Steve, was an orthopedic surgeon. Kim hated to bother him and hated to impose on a friend, so had been putting off Kelley's repeated suggestions to see him.

"Maybe it's stress?" suggested Sara. Both Kelley and Sara knew how stressful the last few months had been for Kim, what with just suspecting and then confirming that her husband, William, had been having an affair with a woman with whom he worked, whose name was Brigid. When Kim confronted William, he had, after much screaming and yelling, agreed to end the relationship with Brigid and had begged Kim to stay with him. Although the relationship had not been rewarding for some time, Kim reluctantly agreed to give it another try. Even though their children were not that young anymore—Patrick was 14, Maria was 17, Eddie was 21 and in college, and Melissa was 24—Kim still knew that a divorce would be very difficult for them. She loved her kids so much that she was willing to put up with a less-than-satisfactory personal life for another few years for their sakes.

Needing someone to talk to, Kim had confided in Sara and Kelley about her anguish and her decision. Their support helped her make it through that difficult time. "Yes, it probably is," admitted Kim. "You know what stress can do."

"Yes, I know what stress can do, but I still think you should have Steve look at it," responded Kelley. "I'm going to have Carol call you and schedule an appointment for him to look at you."

"Oh, no, Kelley . . ." started Kim.

"Come on, Kim, just let him look at it. Do it for me so that I don't worry about you," interrupted Kelley. "You know what stress can do to me, too! Don't make me worry—just let him take a quick look at you."

As Kim groaned and Sara laughed, Kelley nodded and said, "Good, that's settled." Their conversation then turned to Kim's impatiens. Working together, they were able to finish planting the flowers before Patrick and Maria got home.

* * *

Due to a cancellation, Carol, Steve's office administrator, was able to schedule an appointment for Kim the next day. When he returned home that night, Kelley immediately asked how his exam with Kim had gone. Steve explained that the problem was not really in Kim's shoulder—it was in her neck, she was just experiencing the pain in her shoulder. Steve had not been able to isolate the problem specifically, so he referred her to a colleague who specialized in such neck problems, Dr. McMahon.

Having already been concerned about the persistence of Kim's problem, Kelley was even more upset at this news. This defined it for her as much more serious than she had hoped it would be. She called Kim, who again made light of the problem and said, "Oh, I'm sure Sara's right—it's just stress. I may not even keep that appointment with Mc-what's-his-name."

"Don't you dare cancel that appointment, Kim Schmidt! This needs to be attended to!" responded Kelley in concern.

"Okay! Okay! Don't yell at me!" Kim laughed. "I'll go."

* * *

Just to make sure that she did go, Kelley drove her to the appointment a couple of days later. Dr. McMahon, too, was not able to immediately ascertain the problem. Several days and several tests later, the doctor finally concluded that the problem was a cervical disk in the upper spinal cord. He operated and, after a short recovery period, Kim started feeling much better. The next several months went well—still tense at home, but much less painful.

* * *

Several months later, however, Kim started experiencing severe headaches and noticing a loss of feeling in her arms. The headaches she again attributed to stress, but the numbness couldn't be so quickly discounted. She was reluctant to take anything but acetaminophen for the headaches, and was also reluctant, initially, to mention anything about these new problems to Kelley. She did, however, confide in Sara. When Sara, who wasn't one to overreact, seemed alarmed, Kim mentioned the symptoms to Kelley.

"What kind of problem can cause severe headaches?" she began. As Kelley probed more, Kim confessed that she was afraid she had a brain tumor.

Kelley, of course, was immediately concerned and convinced Kim to return to both Steve and Dr. McMahon. At this point, Kim, too, began to acknowledge that she was really worried about her condition. She shared her concerns for the first time with William, her husband, who reassured her that it was probably nothing. He didn't seem to be worried.

Neither Steve nor Dr. McMahon, however, were able to find the cause of Kim's problems. They finally sent her to a neurologist, who also couldn't isolate the problem. By this point the numbness had spread to Kim's leg and her gait was being affected by her dragging leg. The doctors tested her for Parkinson's, Multiple Sclerosis, and a brain tumor, but still found nothing.

The neurologist treated the symptoms with steroids, which helped the numbness but caused such swelling in her face and neck that she wouldn't leave the house. This was difficult for Kim, who was very outgoing and gregarious. She saw only her family and Sara and Kelley. Her children, too, were experiencing the stress of worrying about their mother. Family activities were limited, of course, but Kim tried to convince the kids to continue with their normal activities as much as possible. She felt bad that she was not able to go to events with them, but also felt that her appearance would embarrass them if she did go.

Her appearance did, indeed, seem to bother William. Their sex life, which hadn't been good for some time, dwindled to practically nothing. Although some affection from him would have been reassuring and comforting for her, she felt reluctant to even broach the topic.

She did, however, confide in Sara and Kelley about her loneliness and anxiety. "I know this is going to sound really strange," she began, "but I think that everybody has cancer in their bodies and it emerges sometime when they're under stress. I know I have a tumor—they just can't find it."

Although Sara tried to reassure her and convince her that she wasn't that seriously ill, Kelley responded differently. "I think you could be right, Kim. And I think you're a very brave person to be able to confront it rather than denying the possibility like most people do. The sooner you have it taken care of, the better the odds are."

As time went on, Kim's numbness increased, but repeated CAT scans still showed little. Kim finally ended up in the hospital paralyzed from the neck down. Crying, she grabbed Kelley's hands and begged, "Kelley, please help me! No one's listening to me. They don't think there's really anything wrong with me. They think it's all in my head. They don't believe me! Please help me!" Trying to be strong for her friend, but wanting to cry herself, Kelley promised that she would help.

Kelley immediately went to Steve's office. Catching him in between patients, she shared Kim's plea. As soon as he was through with patients that day, he went to the hospital. He gathered all of Kim's medical records and x-rays, and took them to the radiology reading room. As he carefully pored over them for several hours, he could finally discern some changes over time in her spinal cord indicating some definite paralysis emerging. He still, however, could not find a tumor.

He immediately tried to call Dr. McMahon, but instead was put in contact with Dr. Baase, McMahon's partner, who was on call for him that night. He showed the records and x-rays to Baase, who agreed with Steve's assessment of the situation. By this point, Kim had been moved to intensive care. Steve and Dr. Baase arranged to take her to surgery the next day.

Steve went home late that night and told Kelley, "I think you should go see Kim."

"Is it bad?"

"Yes, I really think you should go see her, if you want to see her again."

Knowing that Steve was not prone to overreaction, Kelley immediately went to the hospital. It was late and Kim had left word that she didn't want to see anyone. She did, however, see Kelley.

"Pray for me," she asked Kelley. "And stay with the kids during my surgery. They're really worried."

Kim, too, was worried—about the surgery itself, her prognosis, and her children. She was especially worried about her oldest son, Eddie, with whom she had not had a very good relationship in recent years. Kim had not approved of some of the lifestyle decisions her son had made, and had ridden him pretty hard about them. They had not been getting along well.

Although Kim wasn't Catholic, she asked Kelley, who was a strong Catholic, to say some Hail Mary's with her. They prayed together into the night.

* * *

Three of Kim's four children—all except the one who was going to school out of state—and her husband were at the hospital early the next morning for the surgery. Kelley sat with them and tried to make small talk some of the time, to reassure them at other times, and to talk about their feelings when it looked like they wanted to do so. Melissa, the oldest, and Patrick, the youngest, seemed to be particularly upset. Dr. Baase did the surgery, but Steve went in with him and updated the family every hour. They found a very, very small tumor *inside* the spinal cord itself. Baase thought that this tumor was causing the paralysis. They were able to remove most of it—enough to take the pressure off the spinal cord for a while. Steve, however, didn't think that they had been able to get all of it.

* * *

Kim's paralysis didn't improve much, but she was able to sit in a chair in her hospital room if someone lifted her into it. After the surgery her spirits were lifted for a while—she was relieved that it hadn't been all in her head and that something had finally been done. However, when she saw that she wasn't getting better, her spirits dropped again. Whereas in the past she had perceived that no one believed her, she now felt that no one was telling her the truth. She begged the doctors and nurses, "Tell me the truth. Tell me what's going on."

No one could or would give her an answer. She told Kelley and Sara, "What, do they think I'm stupid? Do they think I can't handle it? I can tell by how I feel that I'm dying—and I can tell by how they act that they think so, too! Why won't they just tell me?"

After talking with Steve and the other doctors, Kelley still wasn't certain whether they just weren't sure of her prognosis or didn't want to take all of Kim's hope away in the event that the hope itself might have positive benefits. The oncologists urged the family to try both radiation and chemotherapy. When Kim asked, "What are the odds that they will help?" she received only vague answers. Indeed, the entire discussion regarding treatment options was conducted between the physicians and William in front of Kim but without including her. They talked about her as if she wasn't even present.

Without consulting Kim, William elected to try both radiation and chemotherapy. Kim confided in Kelley that she felt extremely dependent and out of control, and that this exclusion from communication and decision making just intensified her feelings.

* * *

One day shortly thereafter, another long-time friend of Kim's, Mollie, stormed into the hospital room. "Why didn't you tell me?" she shouted. "Why didn't you tell me about the tumor? You just told me you were having back problems—not that you had cancer!"

As Kim relayed the encounter to Kelley later that day, she cried, "She was more upset that I hadn't told her than she was that I'm dying!" Kelley was angry at Mollie for causing more pain for Kim rather than trying to support her. Kelley and Mollie were never close again.

* * *

Kelley and Sara continued to try to support Kim's children. They brought dinner over to the house as often as they could. Other neighbors did the same. One evening when Kelley brought a casserole over, she asked for one of her other pans back. William led her to a table covered with about 30 dishes. "I'm sorry," he said, "but I have no idea whose dish is whose. Can you find it?" Both Kelley and Sara thought that William seemed embarrassed at needing and accepting help from others.

Although other friends did try to help William and the kids, they rarely came to visit Kim. When Kelley or Sara suggested to Kim's other friends that they visit her, most came up with an excuse. Some acknowledged, "I don't know what to say to her," or "I just can't handle seeing her like this—it makes me realize just how fragile life, including my own, is." Even the health care providers seemed uncomfortable around her.

* * *

The chemotherapy caused Kim to lose her hair and experience terrible nausea. But it was the radiation that was truly awful. Because they had to target the radiation high up behind her neck, they had to put a conelike instrument into her throat and funnel the radiation back. Her throat and mouth became raw. She couldn't talk or swallow.

"I don't want to go back," she whispered to Kelley and Sara one morning as the nurses were preparing to take her down for another radiation treatment. "It's not helping and I can't stand it again."

"Can't we stop this?" Kelley asked the nurses, who were avoiding eye contact with both Kelley and Kim.

Turning to look at Kelley with tears in her eyes, one nurse responded, "We don't think she should have to go through it, either. But we can't change the doctor's orders. Only her husband or the doctor can do that."

Kelley and Sara talked with William about the radiation and urged him to discontinue it. "She doesn't want this. She should be the one to make the choice. It's her life. Look what she's going through!" pleaded Kelley.

"Mind your own business!" responded William, angrily. "She doesn't know what's best—she's not even lucid most of the time."

Kelley and Sara tried to convince him that she was mentally competent, but to no avail. The older children, too, wanted to discontinue the radiation treatments. Kelley was there with Melissa another day when, upon being prepared for radiation, Kim begged, "Don't let them take me in!" Melissa and Kelley were in tears, but William wouldn't respond to his daughter's pleas either.

Kim's youngest son, Patrick, agreed with his father. Patrick and his mother were very close, and he came to visit her every day. Kelley heard him begging his mother, "Please don't give up! Fight for your life! I'll help you."

Kim knew that she was dying, although no one had told her that she was. Kim told Sara that she could tell she was dying by looking at the faces of those around her. "You can see they have no hope," she claimed. All of the children but Patrick and Maria figured it out, too. Both those who knew and those who didn't know were extremely dissatisfied with the amount of information they received from the hospital staff. The doctor typically visited Kim early in the morning, before any family members were there. He wasn't good about returning their phone calls either. The nurses expressed ignorance about her condition. One day, however, a nurse responded to Maria's question about her mother's chemotherapy with an abrupt, "Well, she's dying, anyway. I don't know why you're even bothering!" Maria was devastated, and stayed away from the hospital for days.

Kim and William never talked about whether she would live or die, although William's insistence on continuing the radiation implied that he thought there was hope. Kim prayed with Kelley and Sara, saying to them, "I know that the end is near. I don't want to die alone. I'm really scared. What if we just die and that's it?"

To calm Kim's fear about what happens after death, Kelley shared with her the details of a near-death experience of her own from a few years earlier. "Remember 3 years ago when I had encephalitis?" Kelley asked her. "There was one night when I gave up. I said, 'I can't do this anymore,' and left my body. I floated up and looked down at my body on the bed, just like you hear people talk about. I finally felt at peace. I was warm and happy. I went through a big, dark tunnel. There was a huge hand there—no body, just a hand. I knew it was God and that he was waiting for me. But I spoke to Mary, because I thought she'd understand. I said, 'Well, OK, if your son wants me, but what on earth will Steve do with all these kids?' That's all I remember, but the next day I felt much better. And now I know that Mary'll be there waiting for me when it is my time."

"Do you think Mary listens to non-Catholics?" Kim asked, with a little smile.

Kelley smiled, too. "I don't know, but I am sure that *someone* does. And you know what else? The next morning, the doctor said, 'We almost lost you last night, didn't we?' He couldn't figure out how I recovered so quickly. But now I know that there *is* something after death—and it's a good something."

Kim never again talked about fearing death and seemed more at peace about her own terminality. She did talk a lot about her past life, however, seemingly trying to make sense out of it and review it.

* * *

Kim's fears now turned to her children. She thought incessantly about the times that they would need her when she would not be there. "They'll have no mother of the bride or groom, no maternal grandmother for their children, no one to call when they just need to talk! I feel like I'm abandoning them." She was especially concerned about Melissa's upcoming wedding. Although Kelley and Sara tried to reassure her that they would be there for her kids, they couldn't take those fears away. Kim knew that they had their own children and would be busy with them. Kim said once, "Well, William will probably remarry. I hope she's good to them." She tried to talk with Melissa about her wedding, marriage, and motherhood, but didn't have the strength to participate in the wedding plans as she would have liked.

Kim also worried about financial arrangements. She had some money, and she wanted to make sure that it went to her children. She didn't feel that she could trust William to do that. So she spent some time sending her daughter back and forth to the bank and the safety deposit box trying to make what arrangements she could.

* * *

Kim finally asked William to take her home so that she could die there, rather than in the hospital. William refused. He claimed, "I don't want you to die in our house. We all have to go on living there. It wouldn't be fair to us to have to think of you dying there every time we walk into a room. We just couldn't handle it. Life is for the living."

Patrick continued to anguish over his mother's prognosis. Kelley could finally stand it no longer. One afternoon, while she was with Kim, Patrick arrived for his daily visit. After he begged his mother to go on living, Kelley gently pulled him aside and quietly told him, "She can't fight anymore, Patrick. She's doing the best she can. She's not going to make it." Kelley then left Patrick and Kim alone and waited in the hall. After a while, Patrick came out of the room. "I feel like she's abandoning me," he told Kelley. Kelley told him about his mother's use of that same word—abandonment—and her fears in that regard. Kelley and Patrick put their arms around each other and sobbed. First Steve and then Sara arrived. Kelley explained to each of them, "I just told him." Neither Steve nor Sara could say a word. There were no clichés or words of encouragement—just silence. They awkwardly patted Patrick and shed some tears of their own. The daughters arrived later, and were relieved to hear that Patrick had been told the truth.

* * *

Shortly thereafter, Kim was taken out of intensive care and sent down to the cancer floor. Radiation and chemotherapy were stopped; she was given comfort measures only. The doctors acknowledged that they hadn't been able to get all of the tumor, and that the chemotherapy and the radiation hadn't killed it, either. The tumor had evidently grown more and was pressing on the spinal cord. Eventually, she would be unable to breathe because of it. The staff knew Kim's prognosis and, for the most part, stayed away from her room. They concentrated on patients who might be cured. There were several times that Kelley had to request that some of Kim's basic needs be addressed.

Kelley noticed some changes in Kim's kids' communication styles at this point. Maria started talking in medical jargon and became very technical about everything. Melissa talked incessantly about anything and everything—except her mother's condition. Eddie, who came back into town whenever possible, changed the topic whenever anything related to his mother came up. All of them, it seemed, tried in one way or another to avoid communication about their mother. When they talked with their mother, they talked about everything except her and her illness.

Kelley, Sara, and the kids would bring tapes of classical music, Kim's favorite, in to play for her, and would read to her. She was aware and would listen in, it appeared, some temporary peace.

Kim didn't talk a lot, but would look at her children as if she was trying to burn a picture of their faces into her memory. It was a searching, anxious look. Kelley tried to get her to talk about it, but didn't receive much response.

Everyone knew, by this point, that it was just a matter of days. They tried to make sure that someone was with her at all times. Kelley and Steve had scheduled a vacation for this week, and anguished about whether or not to go. It couldn't be rescheduled, but Kelley still didn't want to go. Steve convinced her to go anyway—he felt they really needed to get away.

* * *

While Kelley and Steve were gone, Kim went into a coma. The hospital called William and told him that she was dying. They urged him to get the kids together and get to the hospital as quickly as they could. They didn't make it in time—Kim died before they got there. William's first reaction was, "I *knew* she would die before I got there. She had to do just one more thing to make me feel guilty. Like I don't feel bad enough!" Kelley, however, felt that William had deliberately taken his time about getting there because he didn't want to see Kim die.

Kim, however, did not die alone. Another neighbor, Valerie, had snuck into her room late that night. Kim was not especially fond of Valerie—Valerie was loud and somewhat obnoxious—and had requested that she not visit. Kim wanted only her family, Sara, and Kelley with her in those last few days. At first everyone was upset when they heard that Valerie had been there, but they later reconciled themselves to the fact and decided that it was better to have had Valerie there than for Kim to have died alone. The death itself was not a sudden, peaceful experience—it was a long, drawn-out affair.

When the family arrived, the nurses stopped them at the nurses' station. "She just passed away," the head nurse said. The family was taken into Kim's room to see her one last time. After they said their good-byes to her, the nurses took them down the hall to a special room for families of patients who have just died. A social worker joined them there.

Kelley and Steve flew back into town the next day, after Sara called to tell them that Kim had died. At the viewing, the oldest son, Eddie, cried with Kelley, "I know she never approved of me—now she never will! Before, I always had a chance to try to win her approval. That's gone and I'll never get it back." Kelley tried to tell him that Kim had always loved him, no matter what he did. "Then why didn't she tell me that before she died?" Eddie sobbed.

At the funeral, friends tried awkwardly to comfort Kim's children. "I know how you feel—I felt like that when my mom died, too," said an older neighbor to Maria. "Your mother was 73 when she died!" responded Maria, angrily. "She got to see all her children marry—she got to know all her grandchildren. How dare you say you know how I feel?"

Maria was also upset about the euphemisms people used to talk about her mother—"passed away," "gone to a better place," and so on. "Why can't they just say she died?!" Maria said under her breath to Kelley. "That's what happened!"

It was also at the funeral that Kelley found out that a Do-Not-Resuscitate order had been written on Kim's chart without any discussion with the family about it. Although Kelley felt that the order was appropriate, the family was upset that they had not been consulted about it.

* * *

A week and a half after the funeral, Melissa was married. The wedding had been planned for months and everyone decided that it was better to go ahead with it than try to change it. In contrast to the sadness of the funeral, everyone was incredibly happy at the wedding. Kelley felt that they acted like nothing had happened—she felt that they were almost in shock.

* * *

William married Brigid 6 months later. They sold the house and bought another one nearby. The children were all angry at him for a long time afterward, but tried to work through their feelings and maintain a relationship with him. The youngest, Patrick, told Kelley, "He is still our father and he's all we have left. Plus, he's still supporting us. What can we do?" For both Maria and Patrick, however, the grieving period was especially hard. Maria ran away from home during the summer, and returned only when Kelley and Sara found her. Maria stayed at Kelley's house until it was time for her to leave for college in the fall. Patrick suffered from clinical depression for years afterward. He told Sara that he felt his problem was partially caused by how his dad had handled his mom's death. "He always seemed so cold about it. And I could never talk to him about how I felt." And, just as Kim had feared, her children did not get most of the money she had planned for them to get.

The town in which Kim lived and died now has a hospice. It was under construction at the time of Kim's death. Kelley and Sara both volunteer there regularly. As they look at the families around them, they frequently wonder how Kim's death would have been different had the hospice been completed in time for her to spend her last days there. Kelley's mother and father both died in the years following Kim's death, too. They both died in Kelley's home, however. And Kelley and Sara have both written Living Wills, to express their wishes about their medical care when—not if—they are in a situation similar to the situation in which Kim found herself. They both know that the odds are not in their favor and that they had better take whatever control they can now, while they still have a chance.

RELEVANT CONCEPTS

abandonment
advanced directives
avoidance/denial
communication tendencies
death anxiety/euphemisms
personal control
relational conclusion
social support

DISCUSSION QUESTIONS

1. What kinds of social support did Kim and her family receive from each other and from others? How was this helpful or not helpful? What other kinds of support would have been helpful?

2. Was Kelley's confrontation of Kim's illness helpful to Kim? To Patrick? Why or why not?

3. What was effective versus ineffective about William's handling of the situation? About Kim's friends' handling of it?

4. How effectively did the health care providers communicate with Kim and her family? Were there times when Kim and/or her family should have been given more or less information? Why?

5. How much control did Kim have over her situation and how did this affect her? Were there times when she could or should have been allowed more control? If so, when? What impact would this have had?

SUGGESTED READINGS

Ezell, G., Anspaugh, D. J., & Oaks, J. (1987). *Dying and death: From a health and sociological perspective*. Scottsdale, AZ: Gorsuch.

Field, D. (1989). Nurses' accounts of nursing the terminally ill on a coronary care unit. *Intensive Care Nursing, 5*, 114–122.

Kalish, R. A. (1981). *Death, grief, and caring relationships*. Monterey, CA: Brooks/Cole.

Seale, C. (1991). Communication and awareness about death: A study of a random sample of dying people. *Social Science and Medicine, 32*, 943–952.

Sudnow, D. (1967). *Passing on*. Englewood Cliffs, NJ: Prentice-Hall.

17 *Trouble at Laster Enterprises: Managing Alcohol Problems in a Work Environment*

Richard W. Thomas
Central Michigan University

David R. Seibold
University of California, Santa Barbara

TROUBLE AT LASTER: PART I

Recent discussions of problems associated with alcohol abuse have emphasized the increasing importance of interpersonal influence processes in both the intervention and treatment of such ailments (Denzin, 1987; Seibold & Thomas, 1994; Wiseman, 1983). Most important, these discussions have highlighted the significance of viewing alcohol-related communication from a transactional perspective (Thomas & Seibold, 1996). A transactional perspective emphasizes not only the importance of identifying the interpersonal factors that prompt communication and the aims of those messages, but also the challenge of engaging in sequential communication attempts in order to accomplish one's goals (Dillard, 1990). The following scenario explores the role of communication in alcohol-related situations.

Background

Hi. Let me introduce myself. My name is Mark Reynolds and I work as a design engineer for Laster Enterprises. I am 5′8″, 185 pounds, and have light brown hair that is receding at a rate with which I'm not real pleased. But I guess you can't fight genetics. My dad was completely bald when he was 40, so I might as well accept the fact that I will follow in his footsteps (or his hairline steps, as the case may be). I figure I have about another

10 years in which I can comb those strands of hair across my head and at least pretend I am not balding.

When I am not working, I enjoy relaxing on my deck and playing some sports, as long as they don't require much exertion. Fishing, ping-pong, pool, a little bit of softball, and maybe a slow game of tennis seems to suffice. You see, I am not what you would call the athletic type. Although I'm no longer referred to as the "Pillsbury Dough Boy" as I was in high school, I still have a little "bulge" in the front and some slight "love-handles" on the side. All in all, though, I'm pretty comfortable with myself. I like people and I seem to get along with others pretty well. In fact, it was the friendly atmosphere and the people I met that led me to choose to work for Laster. Before I tell you about the problem I'd like you to help me solve, let me give you a little background about the people with whom I work and myself.

I began my career with Laster in 1990, right after I graduated with a BS degree in engineering from Central Missouri State. I wasn't at the top of my class, but my grades were respectable. As I mentioned before, Laster seemed like a really good place to work. I liked the people in my department and my boss, when I saw him, seemed easy to talk to and willing to help me with any problems I encountered.

For the most part, I worked alone in my office. I would do my part for whatever project we were working on and pass it on to the next designer when I was finished. Rarely did I have to work overtime. I knew from my performance appraisals my work was good and that in a few years I would be able to move into a management position. Back then, I felt I had found a company I would be able to stay with until retirement came along. Little did I know what was about to happen.

In 1992, Laster enacted a major structural realignment in response to a loss of market share, due mostly to foreign competition. No longer would we be working alone. Instead, project teams were established and we were expected to work with others from all over the company. For a while, I was scared that I would be 1 of 2,000 to be laid off. I sweated for weeks waiting for the layoff notices. You don't know how relieved I was when my boss finally came into my office one day and said that I had been chosen to work on the Delta team.

In order to prepare us for the change, Laster put us through an intensive training program. Coming from an engineering background, I had virtually no knowledge about how to work in teams. Through a series of seminars, we learned about different facets of group dynamics and decision making, and about the differences we could expect in terms of this new approach as compared to our old way of working. At first it seemed a bit odd, but then I began to see the benefits of this approach to making our company more innovative and customer responsive. We also went through several training exercises with a facilitator in order to help us develop skills in the actual practice of group problem solving. I felt pretty good about myself in these exercises. I realized that I would not be a very outspoken individual in a group context, but that I had the ability to offer important ideas that would contribute to the group's final outcome. The facilitator suggested that I work on my assertiveness skills and not get put off by others who may talk in a more forceful manner. Surprisingly, one of the toughest obstacles for me was calling my new boss by his first name and working with him as an "equal." To me, "Al" had always been Mr. Williams, a person of obvious intelligence and one to be listened to. Now, he was the one listening to me. It took me a little while, but with the help of the facilitator, I was able to feel more comfortable talking and arguing with Al.

Once training was completed, I met my full team, which consisted of two other design engineers, Jeff and Bob, a quality assurance specialist, Susan, and an electrical engineer, Mary. To me, Jeff seemed like an executive, "made to order." Although he had been with the company only a year longer than me, he came across as a very powerful and competent individual. He was 6′2″, about 190 pounds, very athletic looking and, of course, had a full head of wavy brown hair. He was the type of person that everyone paid attention to when he walked into a room. I had always wished that I could be as bold and as personable as Jeff. He was the type of person who could carry on a conversation for hours and make anyone feel comfortable. He definitely had a "presence."

Bob seemed a little shy when I first met him. Bob was about average height (5′7″), a little on the heavy side, and had a quiet voice. I guessed he seemed a little intimidated by Jeff, even though he had been with the company several years longer. However, when I finally got to talk to him one-on-one, Bob seemed very personable and friendly. He said he liked working for Laster but he, too, was a little wary about this new team approach. He said he had always enjoyed working alone and even considered looking for a new job when the team concept was introduced and the layoffs were hanging over our heads. He told me he really stressed out during this period. I don't know, but there seemed to be more going on inside Bob that I couldn't put my finger on. There seemed to be a sadness about him. I don't know if it was the look in his eye or the way he held back talking about himself, but there was something there.

Susan was a lot like me. We were both about the same age and were used to working under the same conditions. She was somewhat short (5′2″) and petite (100 lb) and always brightened the room with her smile. Susan had been with the company since 1987 and she, too, wanted to see these new changes succeed. I think she felt a little uncomfortable on the team at first for, as she said, she had never worked with design engineers before and she felt a little outnumbered. Although a quiet person, I could tell immediately that Susan had a lot to offer the team. She had a more encompassing view of the entire project and a way of cutting through all the surface issues to get at the core problems.

I didn't know it, but Mary and I started work at the same time. However, she had been working in Jeff's department and our paths had never crossed. Mary was a very nice-looking women—5′6″, about 110 pounds, with long black hair—and, like Jeff, fairly athletic looking. On the surface, she seemed a little shy, but very personable and friendly; we seemed to get along from the start. I don't know, but maybe she felt as overwhelmed by Jeff as I did.

Office Party

The project was a tremendous success. Laster had won the contract and was ensured of significant profits for many years to come. As a reward for the teams' efforts, Laster executives authorized a big office party one Friday afternoon. All employees were given the afternoon off and the company provided a big buffet out on the lawn. The atmosphere was exciting. Everyone was "letting go" of the stress we had felt for the past several months and sharing our experiences in this new team environment with our old friends.

At about 4:00 p.m. I caught up with Mary. She had been talking with some of her old buddies and seemed to be having a good time. The party was winding down, so I just sat next to her.

Me: Hey Mary, how are you doing?

Mary: Great. In fact, a little too great, I think. With all this wine, it's easy to forget just how much I've had to drink.

Me: Would you like me to give you a ride home? You're on my way.

Mary: Sure, that would be great. I can get a ride back tomorrow to get my car. Hey, have you seen the others around?

Me: The last time I saw them, they were over at the buffet table. Jeff, as usual, was telling Bob and Susan how the next phase of the project should go. I think they have been enjoying themselves a little too much.

Mary: Yeah, did you see our little Bob. He sure came out of his shell. I never knew what a little wine would do for him. Maybe we should give him a glass before each meeting—it might get him talking more.

Me: Well, between you and me, I think Bob enjoys his wine a little too much. I was eating over at Mabel's the other night and saw him and his wife there. He seemed pretty drunk, and the conversation between him and his wife was not very pleasant, if you know what I mean.

Mary: Wow, I never would have guessed it.

Mary and I walked over to the buffet table. Off to the side, Jeff, Bob, and Susan were going at it in fairly loud voices. It was obvious they were enjoying the party. After seeing them for a while, I was concerned about how much Jeff and Bob had had to drink. Bob's eyes seemed glassy and Jeff was just downing one drink after another. If you can believe it, Jeff was even more loud and obnoxious than usual. I didn't see anyone else paying attention to them, so I knew I had to do something.

Me: Hi, all. Hey Jeff, Bob. Looks like you're having a great time.
Jeff: Hey, buddy. You bet. Here, why don't you join us in a final toast to our success? (Jeff pulled a glass of champagne off a tray from a passing server and handed it to me.) In fact, why don't you come with us? Bob and I are going over to Richie's to continue this party. I think some others are going there, too.
Me: No thanks. I think I'll just go home and get some rest. Besides, I've promised Mary I'd take her home. Hey, Richie's is on my way. Why don't you let me drop you and Bob off there? That way, you won't have to drive. You can grab a cab from the restaurant.
Jeff: Oh, don't worry about it. Besides, I can't leave my car here, and I have to give Susan a ride anyway.
Me: Well, I had planned to come in for a little while tomorrow. I can pick you and Bob up and bring you here.
Jeff: No, we'll be fine. You and Mary should really come with us.
Mary: I'd love to, but I think I've had enough excitement for today.
Me: Jeff, I really think you should let me drive you to the restaurant.
Jeff: Oh, c'mon Mark. Get real. We've only had a few drinks. I've seen you drive in much worse condition. Besides, we're only going a few blocks.
Me: Jeff, please. Let me take you both. We can come back for your car in the morning.
Jeff: Hey, forget it. I said no and I meant no! If you two don't want to come, then don't. But don't give me any hassle.
Susan: Don't worry. I'll take care of these guys. I'll drive.
Jeff: No way, Susie. No one is driving my car!

As Jeff, Susan, and Bob walked away, Mary and I just looked at each other and shrugged our shoulders.

TROUBLE AT LASTER: PART II

Fortunately, nothing happened to Jeff, Susan, or Bob that evening. They came to work on Monday morning acting like long-lost buddies, and except for an occasional snippy remark from Jeff about the incident Friday, nothing was said. However, I could tell that Jeff was not too pleased with me. He appeared very standoffish and it seemed as if he put down any suggestion I had for the team project. In fact, I don't think we ever talked about our personal lives from that point on. We stayed pretty much "on topic" and Jeff and I never again saw each other at any social activity.

Developing Crisis

Over the next 8 or 9 months, our team worked in high gear. We were under a lot of pressure to meet our deadlines and had to work many evenings and weekends. Susan, Mary, and I began to form a close friendship during this time. We worked well together on the job and would spend a lot of time together outside of work. Bob and Jeff were a different story, however. Bob appeared less enthusiastic about the project and preoccupied with other matters. His friendship with Jeff seemed sporadic. Occasionally we would hear about the two of them going out to the bars at night. Also, Bob seemed to be having trouble with the workload and the stress. I don't know what else was going on in his life, but you could tell he wasn't handling it as well as the rest of us. Jeff was still Jeff, very loud and controlling. It became obvious through his stories that he enjoyed his social life. During this period, I emerged as the team leader. Although Jeff still tried to dominate in the group, I became the one who worked to include everyone, to keep the group on topic, and to report the group's work to Al.

It was during these 8 months that the "crisis" developed. As I said earlier, Bob was having problems keeping up with his share of the workload. On several occasions, he missed important deadlines, which hindered our team's ability to stay on schedule. In fact, looking back, there were several incidents that led me to believe our team was in real trouble.

The first incident occurred about 2 months into the first phase of the project. We had to get some design specs to Al so he could pass them along to the Alpha team. During our meetings, everyone said their work was coming along fine and the reports presented at team meetings indicated that we would meet our deadline without any problem. However, at the meeting when we planned to go over all the work together, Bob came in and said he needed a few more days to complete his portion of the project. He apologized for letting us down and said something about problems at home making it difficult to work. Needless to say, we were all surprised and a bit disappointed; Bob had given no clue that a problem existed. I think we were all a little bit angry, too. Jeff looked especially irritated. He said to Bob, "If you'd stop going to the bar every night, you might have some time to do your work." This comment seemed to embarrass Bob, but he didn't say anything. We all agreed to meet on Thursday to finalize the work.

After this meeting, I dropped by Bob's office to talk with him. As I walked into his office, I noticed that his face looked strained and he seemed very anxious.

Me: Hey, Bob, do you mind if we have a short talk?

Bob: Oh, not at all, Mark. I know what you're going to say. I really screwed up today. Look, I'm sorry. It's just that I've had a lot of other things going on and I haven't been able to get as much work done as I hoped to. I promise to have everything completed by Thursday.

Me: Well, Bob, I think you know how important it is for us to meet these deadlines. Just as you need us to complete our work so you can move on, we need you to come through for us. This is especially important since Al is expecting to forward this material to the Alpha team on Friday.

Bob: Yeah, I know. I promise I won't let you down again.

Me: Okay. Listen, I know things have been quite hectic around here. Is there anything I can do to help you out?

Bob: Thanks, but no. It's just that I'm under a lot of pressure at home. You know, the normal stuff—fights about money, work, family. Nothing really important.

Me: Well, listen, if there is anything I can do to help you, let me know. Also, if you want to talk about anything, feel free to drop by.

Bob: Thanks, Mark. I really appreciate it. But I'll be all right.

Over the next 2 days, I could see the stress on Bob's face. However, he did come through for the Thursday meeting. His work was completed and we were able to get our report to Al on time. But I could tell that the rest of the team members were not very happy about the delay. I could see that Jeff wanted to say something nasty to Bob, but I cut him off in time. When we finished the report, we set our plans for the next phase of work. We set up our deadlines and meeting times and I encouraged everyone to let each other know if any delay was forthcoming. Everyone agreed to the process and the meeting ended cordially.

The second incident took place about a month later. I was sitting in my office when Mary came in.

Mary: Mark, can I talk to you a minute?

Me: Sure, Mary. How's everything going with you?

Mary: With me, fine. Except for having to listen to Jeff go on and on about how wonderful he is, I'm really enjoying working with everyone.

Me: Yes, I know Jeff can be overwhelming at times, but he sure does know his stuff. He's made a lot of good contributions to the project. Too bad the way he goes about making them isn't always pleasant to listen to. I only wish he would be more of a team player.

Mary: Tell me about it. Anyway, I wanted to speak to you about Bob. I'm a little worried about him.

Me: I am too. He's been having some trouble at home and it's beginning to effect his work with us. I've talked with him and, so far, it seems like everything is going well. But I'm still a little worried that we'll run into the same type of problem we did last month with the project report.

Mary: Well, I was worried about that too so I stopped in just to have a chat with him this morning over coffee. After a little small talk, I told him how my part of the project was going and asked him if he thought I was on track. He gave me some great suggestions. When I asked him about his own work, though, he seemed to be evasive. He said everything was going well, but when I asked him specifics about the project, he just kept saying everything was fine.

Me: Uh oh. Maybe I should stop by and talk with him again.

Mary: Yes, maybe. But that was not what really worried me. While I was talking with him, I noticed how stressed out he looked. You know, a really drawn face, very tired looking, bloodshot eyes.

Me: Yes, I know. He hasn't been looking good. I think all of the stress around here is getting to him.

Mary: What really concerned me was that I could smell stale liquor on him. It was pretty strong. I know all of us take a drink once in a while, but I mean, his clothes reeked of it. And this is not the first time I've noticed it. In fact, Susan even mentioned something to me about it a few days ago.

Me: Well, let me check in with Bob.

Mary: Thanks, Mark. I really appreciate it. I really like Bob, and I'm concerned about him.

After sitting and thinking about Mary's comments for a while, I walked over to Bob's office.

Me: Hey, Bob. Got a minute?

Bob: Uh, yeah. What can I do for you?

Me: Well, I was just talking with Mary and she told me about all the great ideas you gave her. I think you helped her out a lot.

Bob: Oh, it was my pleasure. I like Mary. She's a really good person and does some great work. I really didn't help her that much. She had everything there. I just pointed out a few things.

Me: Well, I know she really appreciated your help and I wanted you to know. (I also could smell the stale liquor Mary had noted and I noticed how bloodshot his eyes were.) Listen, is there anything I can do to help you? Is everything going okay?

Bob: No, I don't think so. Everything is going pretty well. I think I should have this work ready for the meeting. But I appreciate you asking. If I need anything, I'll be sure to let you know.

Me: How's everything else going in your life? Are things working themselves out at home?

Bob: It's still a bit rough, but I think things will be okay. Once this project is done, I think I'll have more time to deal with the problems.

Me: Okay, Bob. But remember, if you need to talk about anything, please feel free to come to me. I'd be more than happy to listen. Okay?

Bob paused for a second. I could sense that he might want to say something. I didn't want to mention the drinking for fear that it would create more stress, but I wanted to give him an opening if he wanted to talk. However, after a few seconds, he said:

Bob: Yeah, sure Mark. I really appreciate your concern. But I think I can handle this.

Me: Okay, Bob. But please, let me know if there is anything I can do. It's important that we get this work done and not let anything interfere with its completion.

Bob: Yes, I know. I'll see you later.

Over the next several days, I noticed that Bob seemed even more stressed. Our meeting deadline was approaching, and all of us were working intensely to meet it. More troublesome to me was now that Mary had pointed out the smell of liquor, I began noticing it more when I was around Bob. I also began noticing that after lunch (which Bob always took alone), he seemed a little different. He wasn't drunk, but he seemed a little agitated.

With only a week left to complete the project, I started becoming concerned about Bob. He called in sick on Monday, saying that he had the stomach flu. When I asked him if he would still make the deadline, he assured me that he'd be ready for Friday's meeting. On Tuesday, Bob showed up, but looked terrible. His clothes were disheveled and it was obvious that he had had a rough time. His face was pale and his eyes were bloodshot. When I stopped into his office to see if he was all right, he was evasive and agitated. He told me he would be fine if everyone would just leave him to do his work. On Wednesday, Bob called and said he'd be late for work. When I asked him why, all he said was that he had to take care of some legal problem.

On Friday, the crisis came to a head. Jeff and Susan stopped by my office first thing in the morning to let me know they were ready for the meeting. Jeff also commented that he was in no mood to be held up by Bob again. I told them both that, as far as I knew, everything was on schedule and that we should have the report ready to go this afternoon.

At about 8:30 a.m., Bob called and asked if he could talk with me. I told him to come right over. A few minutes later, there was a knock on my door.

Me: Come in, Bob. Have a seat. What can I do for you? (I really didn't have to ask that question. I could easily see that Bob was in a lot of trouble. He looked sick and was visibly shaking. I also detected a strong smell of alcohol on him.)

Bob: Mark, I know the meeting is today, but I'm not ready for it. I know it's inexcusable, but it has been such a tough week. As you know, I was sick earlier in the week and I haven't been feeling good since then. Also, my wife and I had a big fight two nights ago. She threatened to divorce me. I know I shouldn't let my personal life interfere with my work, but this fight really shook me up. I've been up all night trying to get these reports done, but I need a little more time. Is there anyway we could move this meeting to Monday?

I looked at Bob for a second and considered where to go from here.

Me: Yes, Bob, I realize you were sick on Monday. You also said you had some legal problems to take care of on Wednesday which cut into your day. What was that all about, if you don't mind my asking?

Bob: Oh, it was nothing. Tuesday night I went out for a few drinks—you know, just to be alone and to sort things out—and I guess I had one too many. Anyway, I got pulled over by the police. My wife had to come pick me up at the police station, and I had to go back and sign some papers the next morning. Boy, was she mad. I think that's what caused our fight Wednesday night.

Me: Listen, Bob. I don't pretend to know what is going on in your life. All I know is that we have a job to do here. We were depending on you for your work. Without it, the team can't put together its final report. And Al needs that report on his desk at 5:00 p.m. today. Without that report, the entire project is put in jeopardy. Now, this is not the first time we have run into this problem. I thought after our last talk, you would pull things together. In fact, you indicated to me along the way that you had the work under control. You even showed me the preliminary findings last week.

Bob: I know. But it's just a little delay.

Me: Bob. A delay is not acceptable. Al has to meet with the board on Monday morning and this report has to be ready to go today. You know that if we miss this deadline, Laster incurs the costs of the delay. We also run the risk of losing the entire contract!

Bob just looked at the floor. I felt very frustrated and just shook my head. I just wanted to scream. I had no idea how to manage this delay, but I knew now was the time to meet Bob's problem head on. I took a deep breath, tried to calm down, and continued.

Me: Look, Bob. We've been working together for a long time now and I've come to respect your work. But I think there is another issue we need to address here—and that's your drinking. A lot of us around here have noticed that you've been drinking quite often and we feel that it's affecting your work.

Bob: Hey, Mark (a little defensively). I know I take a drink once in a while, and yeah, sometimes I have a little too much, but it's just to deal with the stress. If you were in my shoes, you'd have a drink now and then too. It's not a problem, believe me.

Me: Yes, I think it is a problem, Bob. In fact, I can smell alcohol on you right now.

Bob: Now wait a minute! I told you I was up all night. I didn't even take time to shower or change my clothes. Sure, I had a drink or two last night, but nothing more.

Me: Bob, this is not an isolated incident. We've smelled alcohol on you many times. You come into work hung over and you have difficulty getting through the day. We have had to adjust our schedule for you in the past and now you say you are not ready again. I also believe that you have been having a few drinks at lunch. And now you tell me you've gotten arrested for drunk driving. Don't you see a pattern here?

Bob: No, I don't! What I see is a bunch of hotshots trying to get ahead on my work. I'd like to see some of you deal with what I have to deal with. I just wish everyone would get off my back!

Not wanting to escalate this argument, I decided to back off.

Me: Look, Bob. I don't want to get you angry. I just want you to consider the possibility that your drinking is becoming a problem. Look, I'll talk with Al and see what we should do about the report. Why don't you get back to your work, get as much of it done as you possibly can, and I'll give you a call later today. Okay?

Bob: Yeah, that would be great. Listen, Mark, I didn't mean to snap at you. I'm sorry about what I said. It's just the pressure and all. I really appreciate what you're doing.

Me: Okay, Bob. Let me see what I can do.

After Bob left my office, I called Al and explained to him what was going on. He listened carefully and said he would get back to me within the hour. After talking with the human resources department, he suggested that we meet and get Bob involved in the employee assistance program. He also thought that it would be appropriate to keep Bob employed at Laster, but grant him a leave of absence contingent upon his getting professional help. He said we could not postpone the meeting until Monday. We would just have to go with whatever Bob had finished and hope for the best. He also said that after the report was done, he would like for Bob and me to meet with him in his office.

Wanting to explain this fully to Bob, I decided to go over to his office instead of calling. His door was ajar, so I just knocked and walked in. As I entered the office, I saw Bob put a bottle of liquor in his desk drawer . . .

TROUBLE AT LASTER: PART III

On Monday, Al and I confronted Bob with our concerns. After some initial excuse making, he agreed that he had been drinking too much lately and that maybe it had become a problem. I don't think he saw it as serious as we did. However, with persistence, we got him to agree to take a leave of absence and to seek professional help. At the close of the meeting, he thanked us for our concern. We told him that we wished him well, that we were all pulling for him, and that we looked forward to his return to work.

Recovery: A Month Later

As he walked up the steps, Bob stopped and looked at the Laster building. So much had happened to him in that building over the past year, most of which he wished to forget. Now, coming back to the company after a month of rehabilitation and drying out, he felt scared. He was leaving the comfort and safety of the hospital and his friends in AA, and now had to face the people he had let down. Would they understand? Would they be able to put aside the anger they felt toward him, especially after the last project crisis he had caused? Would he ever be able to regain his own confidence in his abilities? So many questions and so few answers. Everyone at AA said it would take time, and it would not be easy. They promised to be there for him when things got tough, but he was the only one who could begin to set things right and begin to make amends. Now was the moment of truth. He had a meeting with Al this morning, and then with the team. As he continued to walk toward the building, he wondered how it would all go.

The Meeting With Al.

Al: Hi, Bob. It's good to see you. You're looking great! How are you feeling?

Bob: Pretty good, but a little scared.

Al: Yes, I can imagine so. Why don't you have a seat and we'll talk for a while. Would you like a cup of coffee?

Bob: Yes, thank you. That would be nice. Look, I realize I really messed up in the past, and I . . .

Al: Hold on, Bob. Let's just get comfortable first before we get into all of this. I must admit, I'm a little uneasy here too. I've never had to deal with this type of problem before, so I'm really not sure how to proceed. But I want you to know up front that I'll do everything I can to help you get back on your feet.

Bob: Thank's for your concern and support Al . . . and for making this easier for me. I realize now just how serious a problem I had and how I could not have handled it by myself. I know I've hurt my teammates, you, and the company, not to mention my family and myself. I hope that all of you can forgive me and give me another chance. It's not going to be easy, but with your support, I know I can do a good job.

Al: I think so too, Bob. While you've been away, I've done a little reading on the subject of alcoholism and have talked to our human resources people about how our company deals with these situations. I don't pretend to know everything on the subject, but I've come to learn quite a bit. What I think we need to talk about is . . .

Back to the Team. While Bob was meeting with Al, the rest of the team was preparing for Bob's return.

Jeff: I can't believe they're letting him come back. I'd thought they'd fire him. Now we have to welcome him back with open arms, as if nothing has happened.

Me: Hey, Jeff, hold on. Granted, Bob let us down in the past and cost this company quite a bit, but he has a drinking problem. I think we all need to understand what he's been through. After all, it could have happened to anyone of us.

Jeff: Oh, come on, you've got to be kidding. Everyone else here is a professional who knows how to get work done and handle pressure. Bob's a stinking drunk who runs to the bottle at the first sign of trouble. He can't handle pressure, and he sure enough doesn't belong in this company. I've got my career to think about and I'm not going to let him screw up my plans.

Mary: Jeff, you arrogant SOB! I don't think a night goes by that you don't go out and throw down a few. What makes you so special?

Jeff: What makes me special is that I can handle a drink. You don't see me holding back the project, do you? In fact, if it wasn't for me, this whole project would have failed!

Mary: I don't believe you! Are you forgetting the rest of us around here? You may be good at what you do, but without us, you'd be nothing. And, in fact, without Bob's work, you wouldn't have been able to solve that design problem 2 months ago. Remember? Anyway, Bob's dealing with a lot of pressure from home. I think if any of us had to deal with that, we would be sipping a few extra glasses of wine, too.

Jeff: Don't fool yourself. Bob never "sipped" a glass of anything. He chugs it by the gallon. As soon as the pressure builds around here, you watch, he'll be back to his same old drunken self. Christ, he's been sober for only a month, and that's because they didn't have a bar in the hospital. You'll see. He'll be back on the bottle within a week.

Susan: Hold on, you two. This type of arguing isn't going to get us anywhere. Bob's got a problem with drinking and that's the bottom line. It doesn't matter what else is going on in his life. For some reason, he can't drink normally like the rest of us. Now, he's worked hard to deal with his problem and I think we owe it to him to try to help him get back on his feet. Yes, he'll have a lot more to deal with but I don't think we have to add to this troubles. Besides, Jeff, if you knew anything about your benefits, you'd know that insurance covers only 30 days of hospitalization. What Bob needs now is our support.

Jeff: I don't care what any of you say. My career is too important to me. If he doesn't pull his weight . . .

RELEVANT CONCEPTS

alcoholism
enabling behaviors

intervention strategies: direct, indirect, behavioral
problem avoidance
social support
stigmatization
stressors
transactional communication

DISCUSSION QUESTIONS

Part I:

1. What would you suggest Mark do at this point? Should he continue in his efforts? What are the benefits and risks of doing so? What additional strategies could be used in this situation (and by whom) and how might their use affect the relationship between the team members?
2. What elements of the situation and/or the personal characteristics of the participants play a role in how this interaction unfolded? Why is it important to view these types of interactions as transactive?

Part II:

3. Is Bob's drinking behavior under control or does he have a serious problem? What factors enable you to make this determination?
4. What factors led this situation to become a crisis? How could Mark and the others have handled it more effectively and/or prevented it from occurring?

Part III:

5. What are the different ways in which this situation may play itself out? How might the different individuals and the company be affected by what has happened and what will transpire in the meeting, both in the short and long term?
6. How do the different individuals involved view problems associated with alcohol? How do their perceptions of the problem affect the way they communicate with, and about, Bob? How do your perceptions of alcoholism influence communication strategies you would use to deal with someone who has a drinking problem?

REFERENCES/SUGGESTED READINGS

Denzin, N. K. (1987). *The recovering alcoholic.* Newbury Park, CA: Sage.

Dillard, J. P. (1990). A goal-driven model of interpersonal influence. In J. P. Dillard (Ed.), *Seeking compliance: The production of interpersonal influence messages* (pp. 41–56). Scottsdale, AZ: Gorsuch Scarisbrick.

Seibold, D. R., & Thomas, R. W. (1994). Rethinking the role of interpersonal influence processes in alcohol intervention situations. *Journal of Applied Communication Research, 22,* 177–197.

Thomas, R. W., & Seibold, D. R. (1995). Interpersonal influence and alcohol-related interventions in the college environment. *Health Communication, 7,* 93–124.

Thomas, R. W., & Seibold, D. R. (1996). Communicating with alcoholics: A strategic influence approach to personal intervention. In E. B. Ray (Ed.), *Communication and disenfranchisement: Social health issues and implications.* Mahwah, NJ: Lawrence Erlbaum Associates.

Wiseman, J. P. (1983). The "home treatment": The first steps in trying to cope with an alcoholic husband. In D. H. Olson & B. C. Miller (Eds.), *Family studies review yearbook* (Vol. 6, pp. 352–360). Beverly Hills, CA: Sage.

18 *Working With Disabilities: The Case of the Job Finders Club*

Gerianne M. Johnson
San Francisco State University

Terrance L. Albrecht
University of South Florida

The soft *ding* of the elevator door opening onto the fourth floor of the hospital was almost lost in the bustling noises of the outpatient ward. Kim MacDonald stepped off the elevator and trailed Rusty down the corridor past the admitting station. Making a right-hand turn halfway down the corridor, Kim felt a blast of sun from the west-facing windows, turned left, and reached for the brass door handle. This room was reserved for the weekly Job Finders Club meeting.

"So we're the first ones here, eh, Rusty? Sit down, I'll get some windows open." Kim walked the length of the conference table to the windows at the opposite end of the room. There were 10 chairs around the table and 20 or so additional chairs lining the walls. Crossing to the corner to raise the window shade, Kim tripped over an unforeseen obstacle and hit the floor with a crash, wincing at a blow to one shin.

"Ouch!" Kim reached for the corner chair in order to rise without putting weight on the sore leg. Something moved.

"Hurrumph!"

"Excuse me. I had no idea that anyone was using the room. We'll be starting a meeting here in a few minutes. Maybe you could move to one of the other lounges on this floor." This is probably one of the vets waiting for outpatient treatment, Kim thought. He probably dozed off in this deserted lounge. Maybe he's homeless.

"Er, hi. My name's John Salazar. I'm the new custodian assigned to this floor. I'm waiting for, uh, I'm supposed to get a signature for the room. And I'm here for the meeting, too."

Kim stuck out a hand. "My name is Kim MacDonald. I lead the group and I work as a counselor up on the sixth floor. I can sign for the room."

"Okay, I'll go get the form." Yawning and rubbing his eyes, John walked away from Kim and Rusty and out of the room. As the door closed, Kim heard the faint ring of the elevator arriving and the nervous hm-hmm of Howard Latimer, a long-time friend and fellow founding member of the Job Finders Club.

"Howard, come on in." Just behind Howard came the tap-swish, tap-swish of a person walking on crutches. Howard slipped into a chair across the table from Kim but the woman on crutches stopped just inside the door.

"Excuse me. Is this the Job Finders Club?"

Kim reached up from scratching Rusty's ear to offer a handshake.

"Hello, I'm Kim MacDonald, the club leader. We're a support group for anyone with a disability, whether you're looking for work, trying to hold onto a job, or even changing jobs. Come on in."

"Thanks," she replied, and moved forward a step.

"We meet weekly to discuss job search strategies, returning to work, or career mobility issues, based on each member's particular situation and interests."

"It's hard to be mobile in your career when you need health insurance," Howard chimed in.

Kim continued, "Is this the meeting you're looking for?"

"Yes, it is," she replied. "In today's economy beggars can't be choosers. Oh, by the way, I'm Grace de Deur. This is just temporary for me really. My doctor says I have to be on crutches for 8 or 10 weeks. It's quite awful. I had to park almost three blocks from this door and this is a hospital!"

"Huh-hmm, may I assist you?" Howard offered as he rose and pulled a chair out from the table for her. He propped her crutches against the wall. "I'll put these here where you can reach them when you want to get up, okay?"

Grace smiled appreciatively, taking off her leather driving gloves. The diamond ring on her left hand made Howard wonder what she was doing at the Job Finders Club but he was too polite to ask.

Lenore Marcus was the next to open the lounge door. She winced as she released the brass handle and again as she pulled out a chair from the table.

"Ouch!"

"Hi, Lenore." Kim smiled. "It's good to see you." A young man had walked into the room with Lenore, but he sat down in a chair near the door without speaking to anyone. He watched the door anxiously and avoided looking at anyone in the room. Howard cleared his throat nervously.

"Hello," Kim said. "Can I help you?" No answer. "Hello?"

Lenore walked to the door and faced the young man directly. He looked up at her. After a minute, Grace said, "Well, for heaven's sake, someone say something!"

"Are you looking for the Job Finders Club?" Lenore asked the young man. His head bobbed up and down, and he pointed at the door, then to his wristwatch, which read 3:55 p.m. Lenore guessed correctly that he was waiting for someone else to arrive.

As Kim waited for Lenore to say more, the young man gestured with his hands. Lenore knew he was signing letters of the manual alphabet, but she did not know the letters and the gestures were far too fast for her to comprehend. She started to motion with her hand, winced, and stopped.

"Howard, write a note," she said.

"No," Kim interrupted, "just ask if he's waiting for an interpreter." As Lenore and Kim spoke, the man watched their faces intently and he nodded excitedly when Kim said the word *interpreter.*

"Oh, he's waiting for an interpreter," Grace said. "That must be awkward. What if the person doesn't arrive?"

Kim opened a braille wristwatch to check the time. "It's a few minutes past four. Let's get started. We have a small group today, Grace. There are usually at least two other people. We'll see if Max shows up today; he can be unpredictable. Hazel called to say that she will not be here today because of a doctor's appointment. She has to miss our meeting to see her doctor during clinic hours."

Lenore winced. Howard cleared his throat and Grace raised her eyebrows ever so slightly. She tapped one manicured fingernail on the tabletop.

"Who wants to start?" Kim paused. "Grace, would you begin by introducing yourself and telling us how you came to find this group? I'm sure we'd all like to get to know you."

The door opened and John entered. "Excuse me, Kim," he interrupted. "I have a message for someone here named Steve."

"There's no one here by that name," Kim started to say, but Lenore turned to the man near the door and said, "Are you Steve?"

He nodded. Then John said, "A guy called and said he can't make it today, says he's sick." He handed a pink message slip to Steve, who looked crestfallen at first, then angry. He rose and stormed out of the room.

* * *

Steve pushed the button for the elevator and waited, fuming, for the doors to open. "After 20 years of this, I cannot believe I have to rely on other people to communicate in a group. I can't read lips when other people never turn their faces toward me, so I miss half of the conversation," he said to himself.

Steve was congenitally deaf and he had read lips and been fluent in American Sign Language ever since he could remember. He did well in school, even at Gallaudet, but there were still restrictions placed on his communication with nonsigning people, which was practically everyone. Sometimes he wanted to forget everyone he knew who could hear, that is, to give up on everyone but his deaf friends. But for now he needed to find a job to support himself. The elevator opened and he walked in, vowing that he would return to the Job Finders Club for next week's meeting.

* * *

Inside the room, John laid a metal clipboard and pencil on the table next to Kim's outstretched hand. The piece of paper attached to the clipboard had a slightly raised line under the signature space, made out of clear plastic tape. John moved Kim's hand first to the pencil and then to the blank signature line as Kim smiled.

Pretty smooth, Kim thought. He had never met me before I fell over him sleeping in the corner today but he has already adapted to my lack of sight. Pretty impressive.

John walked to the back of the room and moved the big push broom from where it had fallen onto the floor, putting it underneath the row of chairs. Now no one could step on it and fall down. He sat down, yawned, and closed his eyes.

Grace realized she had been staring, first at Kim signing the form, and then at John, who looked as though he was preparing to go back to sleep. This would never be tolerated in a private corporation, she thought. She recovered her composure and checked her watch, wondering if it was still possible to leave or pretend that she had never come to this embarrassing meeting. Then she realized that everyone was looking at her and that they were waiting for her introduction.

"Well, my name is Grace de Deur. I'm a senior manager with a bank here in town. I'm temporarily gimped up by this ski injury." Grace hesitated, realizing that she had said the wrong thing by using the word *gimp*. She hoped no one else had noticed.

"Anyway, I'm temporarily handicapped. I had to have knee surgery and it wasn't successful. So I had to have another operation and the doctors don't know yet if that worked. Between the two operations, I've been walking with these things for 3 months already and I don't know how much longer I'll need them. At least another 8 to 10 weeks. When I heard about your club, I thought that perhaps my experience and contacts in the business community would be of some help to your group." Grace stopped speaking abruptly.

The truth was that the bank president had given her a choice to either attend this meeting or see the company psychiatrist. After her ski injury and subsequent knee operation, she had shown signs of extreme stress that eventually impacted her ability to effectively supervise employees at the bank. The president knew Kim MacDonald and felt that the club might help Grace cope with stress related to her temporary disability. At the very least, he hoped the experience would help Grace put her own circumstances in perspective by comparing them with those of people who have permanent disabilities and quite different career issues than hers.

"It's nice to have you with us, Grace. You're welcome to attend as many meetings as you like. I'm Kim MacDonald. I lead the group and work here in the hospital as a counselor. It's a chance to give something back, I guess." Kim tried to ignore the nagging angry feelings that always seemed to accompany these introductions. Kim's habitual thought, that giving one's eyesight for one's country was more than an adequate contribution for any person to make, managed to surface anyway. Grace looked slightly puzzled.

"Kim stepped on a mine while working in a field hospital in Vietnam," Howard volunteered.

"That was years ago, Howard," Kim responded. "I've worked hard to forget that time in my life, Grace. I spent some pretty unpleasant years in rehab after I got out of the service. I worked in sheltered workshops, had surgeries. I even lived in a hospital like this one, at first. I got through college, at least the BA, with help from the Veteran's Administration."

Of course, Kim thought, the V.A. had been of little help in completing the MA and PhD in counseling psychology. These were not considered attainable career choices for a blind veteran at the time. As a result, Kim received no special assistance or accommodations related to blindness during graduate school, although veteran's benefits still paid for tuition and books. Instead, part-time jobs at the hospital, first in the cafeteria, and later as an orderly on the psychiatric ward, provided Kim's living expenses during graduate school.

"I've been a counselor here for the past 8 years, trying to give something back to the V.A. and to show other vets that they can still have a decent life with, or maybe in spite of, their disability."

"That's incredible, I'm sure," Grace murmured.

Lenore went next. "My name is Lenore Marcus. I'm a data-entry technician, or at least I was a data-entry technician, until I started having repetitive strain injury [RSI]. Now I'm out of work and on worker's compensation. I joined the club last year when this happened. Like you, Grace, I thought it was just temporary for me, too!" She looked straight at Grace. "Wrong! My surgery was 'not successful,' as they say. I'm permanently disabled and suing my employer for negligence and damages."

Grace peered at Lenore, noting that she did not appear to be handicapped in any way. As a senior manager, Grace was all too familiar with the rising number of RSI among employees whose jobs required substantial computer usage. She was also familiar with the absenteeism and turnover data for the bank's night shift, primarily the data-entry technicians. Most of them were college students like Lenore. Grace had the impression that they would fake an illness or injury if a good party came along on a night they were scheduled to work.

Grace asked Lenore, "Were you under the care of a physician at your place of employment?"

"Well, no. I didn't complain when my wrists first starting hurting because, in my line of work, management thinks you're lazy or that you want to make them look bad. I tried to tough it out. Eventually, I could barely sleep at night my wrists were so sore. My productivity dropped and I was seen by a company doctor who recommended that I have the surgery. As it was, I barely made ends meet on my data-entry wages. Now I'm penniless with these disability payments, plus I have a lot of extra bills. Besides that, I'm having a hard time finishing school without being able to use my hands that much. I can't write. I can't carry books. I feel like I'll never get another job."

"That's almost like completing a PhD without being able to see and read the paperwork, right, Kim?" Howard offered.

Kim smiled. "That's right, Howard. Why don't you introduce yourself to Grace?"

"All right. I'm Howard Latimer. I, hm-hmm, work in computer graphics. I joined this group 2 years ago, in fact at the very beginning. I was diagnosed with multiple sclerosis [MS] about 10 years ago. I met Kim here at the hospital. We actually started the Job Finders Club together.

"Of course, I already had a job, the same job I have now," Howard continued. "I'd like to change jobs actually. But, well, there are the health benefits, you never really get those back. At least I would lose a great deal because of exclusionary insurance contracts. Anyway, I get a lot of support from this group. They've helped me deal with a lot."

There was a pause and Kim heard a gentle snore. John had fallen asleep. Kim made a mental note to mention this to the custodial staff supervisor, or better yet, to wait until after everyone else left and then ask John if he was getting enough sleep at home.

The door banged open and Max Madden rolled into the room in a rundown electric wheelchair that had backpacks hanging off the armrests and handles. There was a neon blue SAVE THE WHALES sticker on one of the packs.

"Freaking elevator!" Max muttered as he rammed the arm of the chair into the legs of the conference table. "Sorry I'm late."

Max also was a veteran and member of the Job Finders Club. He severed his spine in a car accident while home on leave from basic military training. Now 34 years old, Max was unemployed, untrained, and unhappy. He was wearing tattered sweatpants and a T-shirt.

"Whom do we have here?" Max asked, giving Grace the once-over. Grace quickly tried to rearrange her facial expression to one of polite neutrality.

"I'm Grace de Deur."

". . . and there go I," Max scoffed.

"Excuse me?" Grace raised an eyebrow.

"Nice to meet you. I'm Max Madden."

"I'm glad you could be with us today, Max," Kim said dryly, suppressing a smile. Kim resolved to talk to Max privately about these late entrances. Today's arrival was more typical than not.

"Where were we? Oh, yes. When we left off last time we were just starting to list the issues we want to discuss during the next month's meetings. Howard, do you have the list?"

"Yes," Howard replied. "We already have mentioned some of these issues again today. Do you want me to read the ones we have written down?"

"Sure."

"Well, first, we said we wanted to talk about how to ask for, and get, what we need at work, meaning reasonable accommodations for our disabilities."

"Yeah!" Lenore interrupted. "I did not know how to tell my supervisor that my wrists were hurting without sounding like a whiner. Data-entry technicians really do need hourly breaks! Can we talk about that?"

"Yes," Kim replied. "When folks used to tell me, 'You can't bring that dog in here,' I wanted to snap, 'Try and stop me!' It's easy to become defensive, or to offend someone else, for that matter."

Grace spoke up. "I know what you mean. People at the bank have been downright insensitive since I've been on crutches. I have trouble getting through that small space behind the counter and some tellers won't move an inch to let me by. If they do move, they make it a big production and it's embarrassing. It makes me angry, too."

"If you want to talk about accommodation, let's talk physical barriers, you know, curbs, doorways, that type of thing," Max retorted. "I had to ride the service elevator with the garbage at my last job. I could never open that big safety gate without help. So I was always waiting for some sucker to help me get up; help me get down. Every trip to the bathroom, every lunch break, and before and after work, I had to have help. I should have sued them."

"Well, I was thinking of more social and political aspects of being accommodated," Howard said.

"What do you mean, Howard?" Kim asked, thinking privately that the issue of physical and architectural access was one of the political hot potatoes of the Americans With Disabilities Act (ADA), one of the most recent and substantial pieces of disability legislation in the United States.

Many initial lawsuits filed under the ADA were grievances about limited physical access.

"Well, hmm, I think the people at my company have started treating me differently over this past year. As my physical capabilities have deteriorated, the special treatment I'm getting from coworkers is not what I want or need. They say things like, 'Howard, don't worry about moving that,' or 'Howard, we'll come to *you,*' meaning all meetings now happen at my office. I protest, but I sometimes feel that they don't respect me professionally the way they once did. And physical strength isn't a qualification for a computer programmer."

"I'm glad you said that, Howard." Lenore spoke up. "I never really know what to say when people ask me what happened to my wrists, or when they asked me how my 'vacation' was after I came back from 2 months off with my surgery. You know, it's not their business but I don't want to be rude either. I do want to know my legal rights. Kim, can we talk about that?"

"Sure, Lenore," Kim responded. "I'm planning to use our next meeting to talk about the ADA because there are some important implications for us with regard to accommodating disabilities in the workplace. Some issues are legally mandated. Those are the things that a company *must* do if they have more than about 20 employees. These are things like making doorways and elevators physically accessible, Max.

"There are other kinds of accommodations that are going to have to be negotiated between employers and employees and, in some cases, in the courts. So far, there are no hard-and-fast rules about which accommodations are reasonable and which aren't. The ADA says that reasonable accommodations should not cause the employer undue hardship. That's generally a financial judgment based on the size of the company, the number of employees, and the estimated cost of the necessary accommodations. The specific details of what constitutes undue hardship are still being determined by the courts. So, for now, the burden of communicating our needs for accommodation remains on us. The better informed we are, and the more effectively we can communicate our needs to employers, the better our chances of being successfully accommodated at work." Kim paused and turned to Lenore.

"Also, you might want to consider whether to even disclose your disability on a job application," Kim said. "If I tell a prospective employer that I am blind, I can benefit from the protection of the ADA and from other legal programs designed to help me get a job. On the other hand, I may be crossed off the list of candidates before I even have an interview. If I don't mention blindness, the employer is likely to feel surprised, and probably defensive, when I do arrive for the interview. Howard, are you getting all this down?"

"Yes. At least I think so, Kim."

"I feel like a freak when I go to a job interview," Max blurted out suddenly. "First of all, I have no choice about disclosing a disability. It's pretty obvious when I roll off the service elevator and into the room. What's even worse is that some people treat my chair, which is part of me, like a piece of furniture. They lean on my armrests or prop a foot on one of my wheels, which makes me furious because it's like I'm invisible, or a visible object, rather than a person." By this time, Max was breathing heavily and, again, Grace wished for the comfort and sanctity of her plush private office at the bank. Anyone ranting and raving like this would never get past her secretary.

"Another thing that really burns me," Max continued, "is when some people expect me to dress for success, you know, the suit and all. Do you have any idea how hard it is to get a leg bag under a suit?"

Grace shifted slightly in her chair and Max gave her an apologetic look.

"I'm sorry, Grace. I forget that most people are shocked by even hearing the words leg bag. Well, it's a daily slice of life for me, babe. If my attendant doesn't show one morning, I could die, or at least drown," Max finished with a chuckle. "I'm using my mom for a weekend attendant as it is now."

"How's that going, Max?" Kim asked.

"She hates it!" Max answered. "Frankly, I've never liked it much myself. She's getting too old to be transferring me from chair to bed, bed to toilet, and back to the chair. I'm scared that she'll hurt herself and I feel somewhat guilty about that. I'm not even going to mention the unique privacy issues involved in this arrangement. Suffice it to say that the last time my girlfriend stayed over, my mom almost died when she showed up in the morning and found us asleep together in bed."

"Hey, hey," Howard said, "you're not a child."

"That's true," Max conceded. "But she's still my mom. She's not some employee that I can tell to mind her own business. If I had the money I'd hire someone, like I do on weekdays. But in order to keep working, I need all the attendant hours I can pay for 5 days a week, for the extra bathing, dressing, fixing lunches, plus other things I need help with, like dry cleaning and shopping. I'm glad my mom can help me this way, and she's really a sweetheart. It's just that it's sometimes hard to tell what role I'm playing and what role she's playing at any given time of day."

"You've raised a number of good issues, Max," Kim said. "The lack of privacy, strain on our closest relationships, and image issues are concerns we can all identify with. We all have to communicate what accommodations we need at work."

Not to mention educating everyone around us to our disability, Kim thought resentfully. "We need to let people know how we want to be treated, what names or terms are acceptable to us, and so on. Most people are still pretty unaware of our issues."

"That's not fair!" protested Lenore.

"What?"

"Why do we have to do everything? Why is it up to me to communicate better so that I can get the breaks I need at work? Why isn't it up to my employer to get education about RSI and make sure that it doesn't happen to another employee?"

"I see your point, Lenore," Howard agreed. "I can really identify with your frustration. No one at my company seemed to have heard of MS before they found out about me. One of my managers even asked me if MS was what *Jerry's kids* was all about!"

"This is a good topic for us to discuss," Kim said. "Howard, check the list, will you? Let's see, we've mentioned reasonable accommodation and the ADA, image issues at work, relationships with coworkers and our family and friends, and educating others about our disabilities. Are there any other items anyone would like to add?"

"I'd like to talk about some disability etiquette issues," Howard said.

"What kind of etiquette issues?" Max asked.

"Well, there are some issues of politeness, I guess. I don't really know what to call them," Howard said. "For example, how can I best accept or decline support when my colleagues offer it at work? For that matter, how can other people offer assistance to someone like me, or to us, if our disability is apparent? But it's more than that too. What about eating in public? I find that restaurants are a nightmare for me since my shaking has gotten worse, and I really dread the obligatory corporate lunch date. How can I deal with it, or get out of it, without losing face?"

"I tried to make the bank move the New Year's Eve party to a different location this year. They were having a cruise on the river. But I wasn't allowed to be on the boat with my crutches," Grace said. "It's not safe, you know, what with the boat rocking. Well, next year I'm going to see that all our people can go to the party. After all, maybe some of them will be on crutches."

"They might even need some other special arrangement," Max added.

"Like what?" Grace asked. Her facial expression changed appreciably and Kim noticed a slightly defensive tone of voice.

"Well, like doors that are big enough for a wheelchair, and accessible bathrooms, and I don't mean one that's 4 miles away from the rest of the party. I'm talking about equal access for all your employees. What about multiple chemical sensitivity [MCS]? I bet you a bank party is one big perfume and cologne festival, isn't it? I mean, people are dressed to the hilt and smelling just as good, right? Do you realize how devastating those smells can be for a person with MCS? And what about the lights? Those twinkling tree lights and fluorescent office bulbs can make a person with MCS physically ill. These people would avoid your party like the plague.

Besides, the people who throw these kinds of parties see it as unreasonable or as an undue hardship to accommodate these special needs."

Grace had stopped looking at Max and everyone in the group had become very quiet.

"It would be nice if the caterers were made aware of people who had special dietary needs," Howard said.

"Thanks, Howard. Good points, Max. Grace, I hope we haven't badgered you with our frank discussion of these issues. We don't often get to talk to a high-ranking manager as a peer in the disability experience. But these are very emotional issues for us and we've experienced a lot of frustration in these different areas. Please stay and talk with me after the meeting, if you'd like. I do hope that you'll join us again in the future."

"I believe I'll at least come back next week," Grace replied.

Kim turned to the group. "I'll get to work on gathering information on the topics we brought up today for our meeting next week."

* * *

After Lenore, Max, and Howard had left the room, Kim asked Grace, "Are you all right? Max can be rather expressive sometimes."

"I'm fine," Grace answered seriously. She was a bit shaken up by the meeting. These people were so unlike her yet they had so much in common. She didn't like the confrontation but she also knew Max and the others were right. Eventually, her knee would get better and she wouldn't need the crutches. But these folks, and many more, weren't that lucky. She vowed to educate the people at the bank and push them to make it a place more sensitive to the needs of anyone with a disability.

* * *

Still seated at the table, Kim scratched Rusty's ears and considered waking John to confront him about his sleeping on the job. But just as Kim rose from the table, John looked up and noticed that everyone had left the room.

"Where'd everyone go? Is your meeting over?" he asked Kim.

"Is this your working time, John? I mean, you're here in the meeting with us and, although you did need to get the signature, you didn't exactly participate in the group. I realize we've never met before and I'm not your supervisor but John, what I'm saying is, are you getting enough sleep at home? Is there some reason you need to hang out here and sleep?"

John revealed that he had been a custodian at the hospital for many years but that he had never progressed in his career because he had narcolepsy, the frequent and uncontrollable desire for sleep. He fell asleep easily and often at work, and his coworkers and supervisors assumed he was lazy, unmotivated, drunk, or incompetent. His performance reviews were poor and he was afraid if he told his boss about his disability, he'd get fired. Finally, John confided to a supervisor who had become a friend and he referred John to the Job Finders Club. But that was the extent of any help he had received.

"Well, it's great to have you here but sleeping through the meeting kind of defeats the purpose. Before our next meeting, let me check into any possible medical treatment for narcolepsy. As soon as I find something out, I'll get back to you. See you next week."

ACKNOWLEDGMENTS

We appreciate input from Paris Johnson in developing the characters and dialogue for this case.

RELEVANT CONCEPTS

advocacy
Americans With Disabilities Act
employment issues
hierarchy of disabilities
image management
network strain
personal control
social support

DISCUSSION QUESTIONS

1. What were your reactions to those who attended the meeting of the Job Finders Club? Why? How do you think each person felt leaving the meeting?

2. The Americans With Disabilities Act of 1990 applies to any qualified individual with a disability who can perform the essential functions of the position, with or without reasonable accommodation. Discuss each member of the Job Finders Club, in the jobs suggested by the case. What accommodations seem "reasonable" for each person?

3. Based on this meeting, what issues can be identified for discussion at subsequent meetings? Prioritize these issues and explain your rationale for your choices.

4. You have been asked to provide a series of communication training and/or development workshops to the members of the Job Finders Club. What communication theories, concepts, or skills should be included and why?

SUGGESTED READINGS

Balcazar, F. E., Seekins, T., Fawcett, S. B., & Hopkins, B. L. (1990). Empowering people with physical disabilities through advocacy skills training. *American Journal of Community Psychology, 18*, 281–296.

Braithwaite, D. O., & Labrecque, D. (1994). Responding to the Americans With Disabilities Act: Contributions of interpersonal communication research and training. *Journal of Applied Communication Research, 22*, 287–294.

Goffman, E. (1963). *Stigma: Notes on the management of spoiled identity.* Englewood Cliffs, NJ: Prentice-Hall.

Johnson, G. M. (1995). Vision, education, and employee empowerment. *Journal of Visual Impairment and Blindness, 89*, 157–160.

Miller, G. (1991). The challenge of upward mobility. *Journal of Visual Impairment and Blindness, 85*, 332–334.

Varley, J. (1978). *The persistence of vision.* New York: Dial Press.

19 *"I Am a Person First": Different Perspectives on the Communication of Persons With Disabilities*[1]

Dawn O. Braithwaite
Arizona State University West

It has become clear in recent years that persons with disabilities are no longer an invisible group. Becoming prominent in the workforce, in the media, and on the political scene, persons with disabilities are "America's last minority" (Condon, 1987). More than any other event, the passage of the Americans With Disabilities Act (ADA) has focused attention on persons with disabilities, who constitute an ever-growing force. However, even federal legislation cannot overcome many of the physical and social challenges associated with being disabled, in which all areas of an individual's life—behavioral, economic, and social—are affected. Even when persons with disabilities do overcome their physical limitations, they still face considerable social barriers in an ablebodied-oriented world. Uncomfortable communication and relationships between ablebodied and disabled persons can erect great roadblocks for persons with disabilities to overcome (Braithwaite, 1990; Braithwaite & Labrecque, 1994).

A review of the literature on disabled persons' communication reveals several different perspectives on disability: as a health issue, as a social stigma, and as a culture. These case studies highlight how disabled individuals' communication with others is affected by the perspective on disability they adopt.

[1]These cases are a composite of the experiences of persons with disabilities found in research interviews conducted by the author. The names of the interviewees have been changed.

Disability as a Health Issue

From the perspective of viewing disability as a health issue, persons with disabilities are considered unhealthy people. Thus, the person who is quadriplegic, has had polio, or has muscular dystrophy is seen as automatically unhealthy. The traditional medical model views health care as primarily a response to a patient's set of physical symptoms (Kreps & Thornton, 1992). The body is seen as a machine that can "break down," "malfunction," or "need restoration." Thus, persons with disabilities, their families, and health professionals concentrate their efforts on the correction, restoration, and maintenance of the body to prime working condition.

Clearly, when a person becomes disabled after an accident or illness, the health care system will play a large role in their lives. There will be a concentration on recovery, physical functioning, and improving the person's physical and psychological health. However, what happens to this view of the person as unhealthy when and if the disability becomes "stabilized" and the person is able to adapt and use physical accommodations to function independently?

Interviews with persons who have visible physical disabilities have shown that most of the participants with more stable conditions view themselves as basically healthy people "whose legs do not work well," for example (Braithwaite, 1990). This suggests a tendency to reject the perspective that disabled bodies are "broken" or in "disrepair" or that persons with disabilities are necessarily unhealthy. However, the medical model perspective is a pervasive one and when physicians, friends, family members, and disabled persons themselves adopt this perspective, it will affect their view of living with a disability, as found in the case of Glenn Singleton.

Glenn Singleton. Glenn Singleton does not remember much about what happened the day of his accident. All he really remembers is the truck coming toward his car across the center divider of the highway. He remembers swerving to miss the truck and his next memory is waking up in the hospital with his wife, June, looking down at him when he awoke. The next few weeks were a blur to Glenn. The pain was terrible. He was told that he would be paralyzed, that he would not walk again. His physician, Dr. Fletcher, told him that they would get him stabilized and home just as efficiently as possible. He told Glenn that he would need three different surgeries "to repair damage resulting from the accident." Glenn seemed to slip in and out of consciousness as days stretched into weeks and months.

Through all this June was a real trooper, as were Glenn's parents, who were retired. They came to the hospital quite often, and stayed for long periods when June had to return to her job at the bank. Glenn was worried about his own job, in fact. His manager had come by and told him not to worry, that everyone at the office was pulling for him. They sent an enormous flower arrangement and a bunch of funny cards that everyone at the district office had signed. A few of his friends from the office came by to visit periodically. When Glenn asked them about things, they cheerfully told him that his accounts were being taken care of and he should "just concentrate on getting fixed up and getting out of the hospital."

Finally, the day to go home had arrived. Glenn had been in the hospital for 4 months. At the end of his stay, he had gained some strength back and had learned how to transfer himself in and out of a wheelchair, how to maneuver around, and he and June had learned about how to care for his basic personal and hygienic needs. He met with a rehabilitation psychologist who talked with him about the process of making the proper adjustments to match the changes that had gone on in his body. He told Glenn that it would be completely normal to feel some anger and resentment and told him he could refer him to a counselor if he felt he needed to do some work on his attitude at some point in the future. As Dr. Fletcher was discharging him from the hospital, he told Glenn, "You are in generally good shape. We have corrected as much of the damage to your body and restored as much functioning as we could." Glenn just wanted to get out of the hospital and get on with his life.

June was thrilled to finally have Glenn coming home. In fact, she could admit now that there were times, early on, that she thought he would not make it. She busied herself with preparations for his homecoming, wanting to do all the right things for him. June had diligently read up on Glenn's disability because she wanted to make sure that she was able to provide competent care for his type of injury and wanted to help Glenn maintain and improve on the strength and level of functioning that he had built up in the hospital. She had a wheelchair ramp built on the side of their 1940s-style house, so he could get in the door. She had rented a hospital-style bed to help Glenn get up and down more easily, and she rearranged the furniture to make sure that he could maneuver his wheelchair around. The biggest project involved having several doorways widened in the house so Glenn could get through them in his wheelchair and having some modifications made in the downstairs bathroom. When all this was done, she went to pick Glenn up at the hospital and bring him home.

The first weeks at home were wonderful for Glenn. It seemed so quiet after all the constant noise in the hospital. While June was at work, his mother stayed with him and she attended to his needs and provided good company for him. They developed a daily routine that was comfortable and predictable. Friends and neighbors stopped by for brief visits and they brought Glenn magazines, more funny cards, and videos. Some of the guys stayed and watched ball games with him. Much of the pain of the injury and surgeries had begun to subside and Glenn was very glad for that.

When Glenn went in for his regular appointments with Dr. Fletcher, or "tune-ups" as the doctor called them, Dr. Fletcher said he was very pleased with Glenn's progress and remarked that he was "mending nicely." Dr. Fletcher gave him an exercise routine to build up his upper-body strength so that he could get around on his own more easily. Glenn wanted as much mobility as he could get and attacked the exercises eagerly.

Glenn began calling into his office on a regular basis as he was worried about his job. He was told not to worry, that his regular accounts were being taken care of. The truth was, his accounts had long been reassigned. Glenn had handled some of their most important accounts and the clients had to be serviced, after all. Management assumed that he would not be able to come back to work, even if he wanted to, and that he would not be able to resume the traveling that went along with his sales position. Management was concerned that, were he to come back to work, Glenn would not project the desired image of the company. Behind closed doors, the president remarked that, "As much as I have always liked Glenn, we have to face that he is now damaged goods and we will not be able to correct the situation." No one wanted to upset Glenn, of course, so they kept his office intact for the time being. He even came into the office a couple of times. People were genuinely excited to see him and between calls and customers they stopped by to say "hello" and find out how he was doing. At the end of his second month at home, there were staff cutbacks in the company and five salespersons, including Glenn, were let go.

Three months after coming home, Glenn didn't feel well. He felt tired, stiff, and listless, so he made an appointment with Dr. Fletcher. The doctor checked him over thoroughly, but could find nothing specifically wrong with him. This made Glenn all the more frustrated. "There must be something wrong," he told June, "maybe an infection from the last surgery or more problems from the accident that they didn't detect yet." He pushed Dr. Fletcher to run more tests, all of which turned up zero. "What more does the guy want me to do?" the doctor thought to himself. "He's going to have to accept that I have repaired all that I can. This is as good as it gets."

Glenn found himself more and more upset. June always seemed to be running around, either for her job or taking care of the house. She never seemed to have time to just be with him. Glenn did know one thing: He was bored with watching TV, bored with his routine, well, just bored with his life. His mother was driving him nuts during the day. Whenever he tried to do something for himself she would say, "Save your strength, son. I can get it for you." He got tired of arguing with her and let her have her way. He wished he could just tell her to stay at home, but, truthfully, he was not sure he would really want to be alone all day. He just did not feel ready to be on his own.

June was frustrated too. She had been knocking herself out for months, trying to care for Glenn, work, run the household, and pay the pile of bills, which was mounting with Glenn out of work. She was dead tired herself and didn't know how much longer she could go on this way. Glenn was becoming increasingly more demanding and less considerate of her needs. He had not been doing his exercises recently and did not seem to be making much progress in getting his strength back. She didn't want to upset him, so she didn't say anything. She just wished she could get him to adjust his attitude. Everything seemed to be a problem with Glenn. She wished the doctor would find out what was wrong with him and get it corrected soon. She realized that she would never have a healthy husband and, for the first time, she had to admit she didn't know how much more she could take.

Disability as a Stigmatizing Condition

As discussed by Goffman (1963), disabilities are one of many "stigmatizing conditions," which are "attributes that are 'deeply discrediting' " (p. 3; see Cline & McKenzie, chap. 15 of this volume, for a discussion of stigma related to women with AIDS). Goffman described how those with stigmatizing conditions accomplish "impression management," the act of presenting the parts of the self they choose to communicate to others. However, relationships may be prevented from developing because of a "stigma barrier" (DeLoach & Greer, 1981), where ablebodied persons are uncomfortable with persons who are disabled. From this perspective, being disabled can be a major source of stress in a relationship between ablebodied and disabled persons and persons who are disabled may use their communication as a way to try to cover up what some have labeled a "spoiled identity" (e.g., Jones et al., 1984).

One danger of covering up a disability is an attempt to "deify normality" (Jones et al., 1984, p. 41), where persons with disabilities become obsessed with trying to appear and behave as they think a "normal" person should (DeLoach & Greer, 1981). Some try to appear nondisabled at all costs and risk compromising their own successful adjustment to living with a disability. DeLoach and Greer gave the example of a disabled college student who wanted to look normal so badly that he would not push his own wheelchair to classes as it would have made his hands and shirtsleeves dirty. The man spent so much effort trying to appear normal that he flunked out of college because he missed too many classes.

Those who take a stigma perspective on disability see persons with disabilities behaving in ways that are more *reactive* than *active*. They act in response to what they perceive others are thinking about them rather than initiating communication and creating the desired impression. Some outcomes when this perspective is adopted by persons with disabilities, their physicians, family members, and others are addressed in the case of Celine Gentry.

Celine Gentry. It was a warm October day and Celine watched the colorful leaves drop from the old oak tree next to her window. It was hard to believe, but her multiple sclerosis (MS) had been diagnosed over a year ago now. Not that the diagnosis had been the beginning, by any means. She had been feeling poorly for almost 2 years before that. She had been to doctors who had told her she had a virus or a reaction to stress. Specialists did not find anything wrong with her. One even prescribed antidepressants and referred her for counseling. She had since learned that MS, a degenerative disease, often took time to detect and this was especially true for women, as some physicians seem to take women's health complaints less seriously. This past year had been especially tough for Celine, as she had seen a significant deterioration in her physical mobility. In fact, she was using a wheelchair almost full time now, although she used her cane when going short distances.

Celine had quit her job as a third-grade teacher last spring. Not that she had really wanted to quit. Sure, she did have to take a few sick days, but she was lucky to have her worst bout with the disease come during Christmas break. She was determined to finish out the year and then have the summer to rest up for fall classes. In late March, her principal stopped by her classroom after school one day. "Celine, how are you feeling?" Celine replied, "Well, Tony, I have been really tired, of course, but otherwise I have been doing OK." Tony sat down facing Celine. "You know, we all admire how you have tried to keep working, Celine, we really do. I think it is really admirable. But let's face it. You are having trouble keeping up with the demands of the job. I know that other teachers have been pulling playground and lunch duties for you and you have been late with reports, and have missed quite a few meetings. All of that is completely understandable given your ill, uh, your condition. Maybe it is time to think about slowing down and taking care of yourself."

Celine felt embarrassed and tears welled up in her yes. "You know, Tony, I have tried hard with the kids and I still think I am a good teacher." "No arguments here, Celine. It is just, well, I have had some parents express their doubts to me. A couple are very uncomfortable with you in the classroom and worry that you would be unable to handle yourself in a crisis. A few have expressed that you can no longer be a good role model for the kids in the spirit of Pinewood Academy. And, well, well, I have had several parents of second-graders ask that their kids not be placed in your class next year." "But, Tony . . ." Tony cut her off and said quietly,

"Look, Celine, we are a private school and depend on our parents' donations just to keep us going. I am under tremendous pressure from the board. Right or wrong, I think it would be best for you to be able to stay at home and take care of yourself. Think about it, OK?"

Celine was angry. "I have knocked myself out for this school and for these kids and their ungrateful parents. Geez, do they have any idea how hard it has been for me to even get out of bed these past few months? This is the thanks I get?" Yet, in the end, she thought maybe they were right. After all, Pinewood's credo explicitly featured a "commitment to healthy minds and bodies." Celine herself had started the after-school exercise program, which included faculty, staff, and students exercising together. Of course, she had not participated in the program for well over 2 years now. Maybe Tony was right. Perhaps she was not a good role model.

Celine was also aware that people were treating her differently these days. Oh, they were certainly helpful and concerned, sure, but she felt distant from her old friends at Pinewood. It was not what they said or did exactly, it was more what they *didn't* do or say. The spring picnic, for example. She had always been the star pitcher of the faculty softball team, but no one even talked about the upcoming game around her. Similarly, the sign-up sheet for the picnic potluck bypassed her too. The office manager seemed surprised when Celine asked to sign up to bring a dish. She would not look Celine in the eye, but said, "Oh, I didn't want to worry you or have you go to any extra trouble. There will be plenty of food—just come and bring yourself." Perhaps the strangest thing was when she first went from using her cane at school to using her wheelchair. Not one person asked her about it or mentioned it at all. She could not help feeling awkward about that and thinking, "If I got a new car, everyone would be asking me about it. But, I come wheeling in and everyone acts like it isn't happening."

As the holidays rolled around, Celine was restless. She didn't feel good, that was for darn sure, and the doctor told her this was just part of the normal cycle of MS. At least Frank and Jenny had invited Celine to their annual Christmas party. They were her close friends, after all, but she was well aware that her social invitations had been dwindling and no longer took being invited for granted. Frank and Jenny's party was a huge annual affair. It was catered, people dressed to the nines, and the good cheer flowed freely. It was also known as a great place to meet people. Celine had dated only once or twice since becoming ill and not at all since her diagnosis. She still felt pretty awkward in social situations, but, "What the heck, I need a night out and maybe it will be fun!"

Celine was clear about one thing—she did not want to roll around the party in her wheelchair. She had seen how people, especially strangers, treated her in the chair. When she came into the room, they would back up, giving her 10 feet on either side to get through—it was embarrassing! "I am not a cruise ship floating in, for goodness' sake," she would think. Other people would ignore her completely. She could catch them looking at her when they thought she was not looking, but then they would turn away, pretending to ignore her. Finally, there were those people who went way out of their way to be nice, too nice. They would get her drinks, hold open the door, attend to her every need. She would smile and say, "Thanks," but inside she felt miserable: "Why can't they just treat me like anyone else?"

Celine spent a great deal of time trying to find just the right outfit. She knew she would be sitting during the evening and clothes that looked great when you were standing often looked really dumpy when sitting down. Finally, she settled on just the right style and a deep forest green color, just right for the holiday. She arranged to arrive early, before any other guests, so that she could station herself in a centrally located, comfortable seat and asked Frank to put away her wheelchair. She even had Frank push her chair into the house, so she wouldn't ruin the manicure she'd had that afternoon. She brought her cane, in case she needed to get up, but she put it behind the chair. Although not as bad as the wheelchair, she always felt that people looked uncomfortable when she walked with her cane. She could hardly blame them—her gait had become more uneven and she could see how people might be concerned that she'd fall. Well, not tonight. For one night, at least, she didn't have to let her disability be the first thing people saw about her.

It was a lovely party. There must have been almost 100 people in attendance and everyone seemed to be having a great time. Jenny discreetly kept Celine supplied with food and drink without making any big deal out of it, bless her. A couple of men asked her to dance, but Celine declined politely. She didn't say she couldn't dance, she just said thanks, but she was waiting for her boyfriend. She did enjoy talking to a few college friends who she had not seen in a while. One old friend, Brenda, had heard about the MS and knew that Celine had quit her job last spring. "How wonderful for you!" she chirped brightly. "Half the days I wish I could retire. I've been promoted, you know, and I work so many hours I don't have any time for myself! You must be doing all those things you had been putting off for years!" "Yeah, right, Brenda," Celine retorted sarcastically, "I painted the house in June, took up skydiving in August, and in January I am going on safari!" Brenda stared at her and then laughed. "Oh Celine, you have always been such a riot!" Brenda flounced off toward a group of men.

Celine was getting stiff after sitting for several hours. Her neck hurt from looking up at people all night as she talked with them. But she was having a good time overall. She saw an attractive man looking at her from across the room. He looked strangely familiar, but she couldn't place him. She watched him refill his glass of wine and make his way over to her. Celine felt instantly nervous. She had never been particularly shy, but since the MS, she found it harder to meet new people. She was afraid that they would feel sorry for her or be uncomfortable around her. "Oh, no, here he comes," she thought. Alberto introduced himself and asked if he could sit down. Celine said, "Please do," and was very glad not to have to look up to talk with him.

Unlike most new people, Alberto seemed very easy to talk with. He was an engineer and they discovered they had attended the same university. After a couple minutes of conversation, Alberto said, "You don't remember me, do you?" Celine replied, "Well, I do think you look familiar, but, I am sorry I can't place you." "You were my son's teacher at Pinewood last year, James Sanchez." Celine exclaimed, "Jimmy! What a wonderful little boy! I am sorry that I do not remember meeting you, Alberto!" "Well, it was only one time at the Pinewood annual picnic. My ex-wife has Jimmy on most weekdays, so you probably had most of the contact with her." Celine was glad to hear he was not married. "Jimmy talked about you all the time," Alberto said. "You really helped to bring him out of his shell. I heard about your illness and I was sorry when you left the school. I think it was a real loss for Pinewood."

Celine and Alberto talked for over an hour. She was surprised how the time flew by. Unlike most people, he did not ask her about the MS, which was a real change. She offered a few details about it in the course of their conversation, but didn't feel as if she had to. Alberto refilled her wineglass for her, without making a big deal of it. They were so engrossed in conversation, next thing she knew, the party had really emptied out. "Well, I had best get going before Jen and Frank throw me out," she said rather regretfully. "Do you need a ride home?" he asked. She accepted. She felt around behind the chair for her cane and finally had to ask Alberto to help her reach it. As she stood up, she thought, "Well, here goes. Now he'll see the real me." She felt a bit chagrined as Frank brought out her wheelchair for her. She kept watching Alberto, expecting him to look uncomfortable, but he didn't. As they left the party she thought to herself, "Perhaps there's hope after all."

Disability as a Culture

A third perspective scholars have been exploring in recent years is viewing disability as a culture (Braithwaite, 1990, 1996). This perspective views adjusting to disability as a process of assimilating to a new culture. Although a newly disabled person has many physical adaptations to make, the social adjustments are perhaps even more challenging, as the person is usually not aware of the changes in their relationships awaiting them.

DeLoach and Greer (1981) described a three-phase model of adjustment to disability: stigma isolation, stigma recognition, and stigma incorporation.

Stigma isolation describes the adjustment period following disablement. During this phase, the person views things happening to him or her as separate from the disability, for example, not recognizing that old friends are drifting away because they are uncomfortable around the person with the disability. If they are to successfully socialize in their new role, they enter the stigma recognition phase and develop ways to sidestep or minimize the effects of their disability. This second phase begins the process of becoming part of the disabled culture by first recognizing the existence of the culture and by starting to assimilate into it (Braithwaite, 1990).

The third phase, stigma incorporation, involves integrating the disability into the person's own definition of self and developing ways to overcome negative aspects of being disabled (DeLoach & Greer, 1981). Studies reveal that stigma incorporation occurs when persons with disabilities are able to develop communication strategies that allow them to successfully function in the ablebodied-oriented world (Braithwaite, 1990). At this point, the person who is disabled has assimilated into the disabled culture; that is, having a disability is part of their definition of self and they are developing ways to adapt their communication behaviors to overcome potential problems of communicating with persons who are ablebodied. Adopting this perspective impacts the behavior of the person with the disability as well as all those she or he interacts with, as shown in the case of Marcy Monroe.

Marcy Monroe. Marcy maneuvered her wheelchair closer to the bed. The woman in the bed turned away. "I don't want to talk to you right now. Maybe later, but not now." "I understand," said Marcy. "I'm leaving my card here for you. Call me anytime." "In case you hadn't noticed, I can't even pick the damn card up!" the woman exclaimed sarcastically. "I know," said Marcy gently. "Just call when you're ready." Marcy left the hospital. "Whew! Was I that angry? Yeah, I probably was," she said to herself.

Dr. McDowell had been calling on Marcy for over 5 years now. Dr. McDowell was a rehabilitation psychologist at University Hospitals and found that it was often very helpful to have persons with spinal cord injuries come and talk to those who found themselves in the same predicament. Marcy was glad to do it—most days—and remembered how helpful Terry had been when Dr. McDowell was treating her after her accident. Coming here reminded her of how far she had come. There was so much to adjust to.

Marcy remembers Dr. McDowell telling her that she would be quadriplegic. Fortunately, she would have some use of her hands. With hard work, she would be able to maneuver a wheelchair, write, type, and use eating utensils with the help of a brace, and with surgery she would be able to develop enough pressure in her hands to be able to drive. All of what the doctor said had come true. The hard work part was certainly true too. Marcy recalled the early period after her accident. She felt lousy, of course, but was sure that the injury was not as bad as they said. She had never been afraid of a fight and she would beat this thing. Her friends and family came to see her and she tried to be upbeat. "I'll be back in the saddle sooner than you think," she'd say. "Just don't let them give away my locker at the gym!" Her friends would laugh with her and say, "You bet, Marcy!" but no one really believed it.

Weeks stretched into months. Marcy spent time in rehabilitation building up her strength and learning about self-care and mobility. In June, Marcy decided it was time to go home. She had realized that her condition was indeed permanent, but she was not going to let that stop her. In fact, she planned to resume her studies at the university in the fall. She would just change her major to something that would accommodate her new lifestyle—she was not sure what that would be, but she would figure it out later. While she was in the hospital, her parents had closed out her apartment, understandably, and Marcy decided she could live at home for a while.

Home life was not going well. Marcy had lived out on her own for 3 years, and all her freedom and independence was now gone. Marcy's parents babied her at every turn, wanting her to "save her strength." Physically, the adjustments were hard. The house was not as convenient as the hospital had been and, even though her parents had some modifications made, even the simple things like turning on the television, answering the phone, and getting around the house were difficult. Going out was a huge production in itself and it became easier to stay at home sometimes. Marcy came to realize that one part of being disabled was simply time—everything took so much time. For example, getting up, washed, and dressed in the morning, all with her mother's help, of course, seemed to take forever. Marcy longed for the days when she could roll out of bed, throw on a pair of jeans, and be off to school in a matter of minutes. She began to realize that, in her present state, school in the fall would be out of the question.

Something else was bothering Marcy. Her friends, her *so-called* friends, were really being jerks. They came and visited a lot when she was first in the hospital. They were cheery and upbeat. Soon, however, the visits started to dwindle. When she called them, they didn't seem to have much to talk about. Her contact with her friends was now pretty rare. From her friends' side of it, they just didn't know what to do. Fran worried that if she talked about going to a dance or about other activities Marcy was missing, Marcy would feel depressed or left out. Theo and Marcy had started dating somewhat seriously before the accident, but he felt really awkward about it all now. It was hard to know what to say and he certainly didn't want to upset her. She was still an attractive woman, but—and he felt really guilty about thinking this—he didn't want to go out with a quadriplegic. It is just not how he envisioned his life.

Finally, Marcy had a huge fight with her mother about going back to school. Mom wanted her to wait a semester until she felt stronger and could get around better. That was the last straw. Marcy's whole life felt out of control—her body, her home life, her social life—well, her life was not *hers* anymore. It felt like one of those movies when the person wakes up in the same place with the same people, but everything is somehow changed and they don't know anyone or even who they are. It reminded her of traveling in a new country, when you don't quite know how things work or what you are supposed to say or do. She felt isolated and completely frustrated.

One day, she got a call from Terry; Dr. McDowell had arranged for her to visit Marcy in the hospital. "How does she do it?" Marcy wondered. Terry was a graduate student in psychology at the university. She seemed to have her life all together, had her own apartment, and had someone who helped her with daily tasks. Terry even drove her own van and picked Marcy up to go to lunch. Terry laughed when Marcy told her all that had been going on. "Geez, Marcy, you do sound like you have had it. But, you know, even though no two people go through this experience the exact same way, actually, my feelings were pretty similar to yours." Three hours flew by and Terry and Marcy talked and talked. Terry put Marcy in touch with the Center for Independent Living.

The Center made all the difference. Marcy learned about obtaining attendant care, hiring a person to help meet her physical and mobility needs. Once she had an attendant, she moved into a handicapped-accessible building downtown. Her parents seemed skeptical at first, but they relented and now only called every few days rather than two or three times a day. It was not the greatest building, but it was clean and it was nice to have a place that was designed to meet her needs. Also, she was around other disabled people for the first time, really. It was kind of strange at first—she really didn't know what to say to them. When she thought of it, it made sense; after all *she* was the first disabled person she had ever known! After a month Marcy joined a group of women from the building who met weekly. Much of the talk was social and some was about political action issues. It was just nice to have other people to talk with who had similar experiences to hers. The women talked about men and dating at length. Marcy had never realized it, but disabled men are much more likely to date and marry ablebodied women than disabled women are likely to get involved with ablebodied men. The women discussed their own reading of this fact and talked about other issues of dating life and sexuality. And they laughed *a lot*. The humor was often raucous and sometimes downright lewd. All this felt great, as Marcy realized that she had not done much laughing since her accident.

Marcy decided to go back to the university and major in social work. She thought that she had the kind of life experience that would make her a good help to others in need. Terry helped her get registered for classes and put her in touch with the Disability Resource Center on campus. Although Marcy resisted the idea of going to the Disability Resource Center office at first, she soon found out that there were many services available to her that would be very helpful. For example, the Center provided funds for a note taker in each of her classes, assistance in the library with getting books off the shelves, and helped with anticipating other tasks that would be difficult for Marcy.

Having an attendant was very different for Marcy. On the one hand, it gave her the assistance she needed and also the independence from her parents that she craved. As much as she loved her parents and appreciated all they had done, she knew she had to make it on her own. At first, she had a couple of attendants who seemed to want to "run the show." As she talked to other people in her building, she realized that *she* needed to be in charge. These were not friends or family; these people were professionals and her employees. Armed with that mind-set, she interviewed attendants and chose a person to work *for* her.

The other issue with attendants that really got to her was that many ablebodied people would talk to her attendant rather than to her. It was very common for Marcy to have a waiter or a store clerk turn to her attendant and say, "And what would *she* like?" Marcy instructed her attendant to let her answer the question. "I would like a size 10," Marcy told one sales clerk. The clerk looked at the attendant and said, "And what color would she like?" "Blue," said Marcy, now irritated. She moved her chair closer to the clerk and her attendant stepped back. "I would like to look at the blue sweater in a size 10, please," she said emphatically. The embarrassed clerk blushed and mumbled an apology. Marcy felt good about how she handled the situation. It was irritating and this seemed like a never-ending battle, but she felt she could take care of herself. What was it that she wanted from others? Just to be treated like anyone else, that was all.

Marcy also realized that she felt much more confident and able to handle herself than she had earlier. She was working on a group project in one class and could tell that a couple of the group members seemed uncomfortable around her. They would not look at her, seemed hesitant around her, and did not seem to think that she would pull her weight in the group. This kind of thing used to really worry her, but she had come to expect it and had developed ways to work around most people's discomfort. Jim, the worst offender, would ask for volunteers, but would never look at Marcy. So, Marcy made it a point to arrive early, be ready for the meetings, and to offer to do tasks before anyone had to ask for volunteers. She also made a lot of jokes, often at her own expense. At first, this seemed to make some of the group members even more uncomfortable, but soon they were laughing along with her and teasing her. Marcy counted it a personal triumph when Jim started teasing her about having tire marks on her hands and Marcy laughed and said, "If you don't watch it you'll have tire prints across your back!" Finally she felt as if she was fitting in, just like any other group member.

Marcy also knew from personal experience that others were naturally curious about her disability and about what she could and could not do. Of course, most people hardly ever came right out and asked her. So, she would work information into the conversation. "Of course, before I broke my neck, you couldn't get me into the library! But now I enjoy spending time there and have really found I have a knack for research, that is, when I have an assistant there to get those books off the high shelves for me!" When she met new people, she often steered the conversation away from disability for a while. She would talk about music, NBA basketball, or events in the news. Anything to help the other person see that she was a "normal" person and wanted to be treated that way. Somehow, if they talked about her disability too soon, she found that the ablebodied person could never start to treat her normally.

The phone rang and it was Dr. McDowell. "Marcy, you remember that woman I asked you to visit in rehab a few weeks back? Well, I think that she would really like to talk to someone who has gone through this whole mess. Would you be willing to give her another chance?" "Sure," Marcy said. "She just didn't seem ready at that time. I understand how that goes and didn't want to push her." Marcy thought about what she could tell the woman. Although no one could fully prepare her for what was in store for her, Marcy realized that there was much that she could offer. Most important, perhaps, was just to treat her *as a person*. She probably was not getting much of that in her life right now and Marcy knew from firsthand experience just how important that was.

EPILOGUE: TREAT ME AS A "PERSON FIRST"

As I have talked with persons who have disabilities, one central goal of their communication is clear: to be accepted as and treated as "*persons first*," rather than to be treated like an object, as a "disability." This theme of wanting to be personified, rather than objectified, to be treated as normal, to be "treated like anybody else" has been repeated time and time again in the interviews. Participants sometimes discussed strategies they would use in reaction to the discomfort of ablebodied others, but most often discussed communication strategies that are proactive rather than reactive, that is, designed to create the desired impression right from the start of the relationship. The ability to communicate in this way is most often part of a developmental process that usually occurs as a person adjusts to their disability and develops effective ways to communicate with ablebodied others. Viewing people with disabilities as unhealthy or stigmatized promotes a view that many people with disabilities reject, both for themselves and from others. This perspective seems very different than deifying normality and there is every reason to believe that persons with disabilities can come to accept being disabled and also find ways to proactively communicate to create the desired impression of themselves to others. When we look at adjusting to a disability as analogous to assimilating into a different culture, we can focus on how persons with disabilities develop ways to communicate most effectively to meet their goal of being accepted and treated as a person.

RELEVANT CONCEPTS

cultural assimilation
deify normality
health perspectives
medical model
personifying versus objectifying
phases of adjustment
social stigma

DISCUSSION QUESTIONS

1. How is behavior affected when the medical model view of disability is adopted?
2. What are the implications for a person with a disability to "deify normality"?
3. How is behavior affected when a stigma view on disability is adopted?
4. How is becoming disabled similar to assimilating to a new culture?
5. How can ablebodied persons communicate with persons with disabilities in such a way as to treat them as "persons first"?

REFERENCES/SUGGESTED READINGS

Braithwaite, D. O. (1990). From majority to minority: An analysis of cultural change from ablebodied to disabled. *International Journal of Intercultural Relations, 14*, 465–483.

Braithwaite, D. O. (1996). Persons first: Expanding communicative choices by persons with disabilities. In E. B. Ray (Ed.), *Communication and disenfranchisement: Social health issues and implications*. Mahwah, NJ: Lawrence Erlbaum Associates.

Braithwaite, D. O., & Labrecque, D. (1994). Responding to the Americans With Disabilities Act: Contributions of interpersonal communication research and training. *Journal of Applied Communication Research, 22*(3), 287–294.

Condon, S. G. (1987, April). Hiring the handicapped confronts cultural uneasiness. *Personnel Journal*, pp. 28–38.

DeLoach, C., & Greer, B. G. (1981). *Adjustment to severe disability*. New York: McGraw-Hill.

Goffman, E. (1963). *Stigma: Notes on the management of spoiled identity*. Englewood Cliffs, NJ: Prentice-Hall.

Jones, E. E., Farina, A., Hastorf, A. H., Markus, H., Miller, D. T., & Scott, R. A. (1984). *Social stigma: The psychology of marked relationships*. New York: Freeman.

Kreps, G., & Thornton, B. C. (1992). *Health communication: Theory and practice* (2nd ed.). Prospect Heights, IL: Waveland.

Author Index

Subject Index